# countdown to baby

# countdown to baby

*a day-by-day journal for moms to be*

Aimee Chase

**HARLEQUIN®**

Countdown to Baby: A Day-By-Day Journal For Moms to Be

ISBN-10: 0-373-89221-7
ISBN-13: 978-0-373-89221-1

© 2009 by Hollan Publishing, Inc.
100 Cummings Center, Suite 123A
Beverly, MA 01915

The ideas, procedures, and suggestions contained in this book are not intended as a
substitute for consulting with your physician.  All matters regarding your health require
medical supervision.

www.eharlequin.com

Printed in U.S.A.

To my sons, for making pregnancy worth the journey

# Introduction

It is always a miracle when a baby is conceived and begins its extraordinary growth process within the secret confines of the womb. But what's even more of a miracle is how any woman survives the bizarre twists and turns of the 266-day roller coaster ride that follows. When else but in pregnancy is it "normal" to have emotional meltdowns, frequent heartburn, raging acne, leaking breasts, insatiable hunger, and a human being twisting about in your abdomen? And yet, you can expect to gain more than extra weight during pregnancy—you get a whole new respect for your body and its ability to grow a human being; a stronger connection to the person who helped you create your baby; and a deeper level of fulfillment as you cross into the realm of parenthood. *Countdown to Baby* will help you survive this peculiar, emotional, life-altering journey by highlighting your accomplishments as your pregnancy progresses and enabling you to take an active role every step of the way. Each new day brings an update on your baby's growth, insight regarding the changes happening to your own body, and tips for keeping both you and baby as happy and healthy as possible.

*Countdown to Baby* is more than a guide—it's a personal diary; an opportunity to describe your experience of pregnancy so you can track patterns and symptoms, release frustrations or concerns, and build a keepsake of this unique time in your life. *Countdown to Baby* rewards you with new insight and helps you look forward to each day of your remarkable countdown from Day 266 (conception) to Day 1 (your baby's due date)! Savor the highs and lows as you edge closer and closer to the moment that makes it all worthwhile—meeting your baby for the first time.

# How to Use This Journal

Your doctor or midwife should give you a due date at your first prenatal appointment. Enter this date in the space provided at the back of the book next to Day 1. Use a calendar to fill in the rest of the dates working backward to Day 266 (conception). While this journal begins on the day your child was conceived, your medical provider will date your pregnancy from the first day of your last menstrual period (LMP), which is about two weeks earlier. To eliminate any confusion, both forms of measurement (Gestational Week and LMP Week) are provided. The first two weeks of this journal describe events that happened before you even knew you were pregnant. Space is provided to describe how you remember feeling in those very early weeks of pregnancy. If you don't remember how you felt, start your personal entries on that unforgettable day when you found out that you were pregnant.

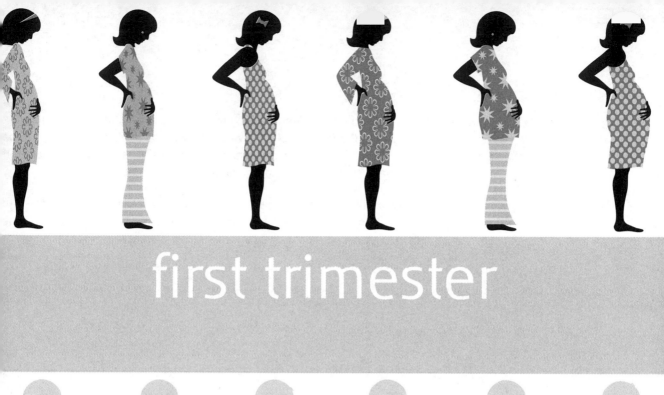

first trimester

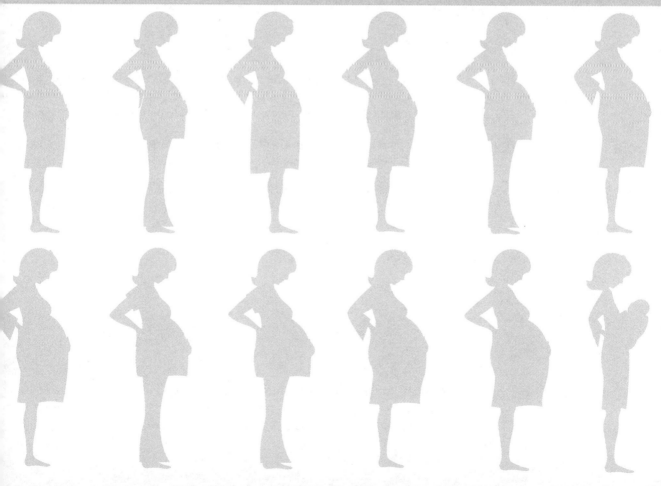

# Day 266 Date_____

**Your baby on this day**

On this day, one of two hundred million possible sperm won the race to your fertile egg and formed the unique cell that would be your baby! Your baby's hair color, eye color, personality tendencies, and more were established when 23 of your chromosomes combined with 23 of the father's chromosomes.

**Your body on this day**

Your fallopian tube may have been hosting a biological miracle on this day, but your body was keeping it hush-hush. Telltale signs like sore breasts, menstrual-type cramping, nausea, and other classic symptoms of pregnancy were yet to come.

How I Feel _____

_____

My Thoughts _____

# Day 265 Date_____

**Your baby on this day**

Your single-celled baby got a little more complicated on this day. He or she divided into two cells. These cells will continue to divide about once every twenty-four hours until they eventually make up all the intricate parts of your baby's body.

**Your body on this day**

On this day your body was clever enough to manufacture a special protein called EPF, which prevents your baby from being perceived as a foreign object by your body.

How I Feel _____

_____

My Thoughts _____

_____

# Day 264 Date_____

**Your baby on this day**

Your baby stayed about the same size on this day, but divided into more cells and began moving slowly down the fallopian tube towards your uterus. There she will "set up camp" and will remain until the end of your pregnancy.

**Your body on this day**

If, like many women, you needed the help of in vitro fertilization to get pregnant, today was most likely the day when a predetermined number of your successfully fertilized eggs (embryos) were inserted into your womb.

How I Feel _____

_____

My Thoughts _____

_____

## Day 263 Date_____

**Your baby on this day**

Your baby was made up of about sixteen cells on this day. He or she was entering or was just about to enter the uterus at this time.

**Your body on this day**

Thanks to a hormone increase in your body, layers of soft tissue began to line your uterus on this day to prepare for your baby's arrival.

How I Feel _____

_____

My Thoughts _____

_____

## Day 262 Date_____

**Your baby on this day**

Your child was still too small at this time to be seen by the human eye, but he would soon grow rapidly in size. He was just starting to make a home for himself in the upper curve of your uterus.

**Your body on this day**

Within about 24 hours of his life, your baby released a hormone called hCG (human Chorionic Gonadotropin) into your bloodstream. HCG told your body to stop menstruating and alerted you that you were pregnant (your pregnancy test was positive because of the hCG it found in your urine). In a way, your baby was already communicating with you.

Week 1 Weigh-in:_____lbs

My Thoughts

> I woke up at 4 am one morning and—I don't know how I knew, but—I just knew I was pregnant. I flew out of bed, ran downstairs, and took a home pregnancy test. When I woke my husband to tell him the news, he was still half asleep. We both just sat up in bed and stared at the test for a while.
>
> –Mia O., mother of 1-year-old Thomas

## Day 261  Date_____

**Your baby on this day**

The new bundle of cells in your uterus divided into two distinct parts on this day. The inner part would grow into your baby while the outer cells would go off on their own to become the baby's support system.

**Your body on this day**

As your baby burrowed into your soft uterine lining, some of the uterine tissue may have sloughed off. This may have caused spotting, a sign that might have led you to wonder if you were pregnant.

How I Feel

My Thoughts

## Day 260 Date_____

**Your baby on this day**

Women under age 35 have a higher chance of conceiving fraternal twins. If you are now pregnant with fraternal twins, two little embryos embedded themselves in your uterus today.

**Your body on this day**

Your blood volume started increasing even before this day to help provide additional blood to your baby, your uterus, and what will soon be the placenta. You may remember feeling faint as a result of this early drop in your blood pressure.

How I Feel _____

_____

_____

My Thoughts _____

_____

_____

_____

*Before I Knew I Was Pregnant*

Gestational Week 2, LMP Week 4

## Day 259 Date_____

**Your baby on this day**

Your baby's cells migrated into three distinct layers, all with separate missions. The first layer's mission was to form your baby's brain, spinal cord, nerves and skin.

**Your body on this day**

Your uterine tissue committed a motherly act on this day and formed a protective cocoon over your baby's body and support system.

How I Feel _____

_____

_____

My Thoughts _____

_____

_____

_____

Week 2 Weigh-in:____lbs

# Day 258 Date _____

**Your baby on this day**

On this day your baby's body consisted of three layers of cells shaped a bit like a shield. Broad at the top and narrow at the bottom—this was the shape of your 8-day-old baby.

**Your body on this day**

Knowing you were pregnant, you body started conserving more iron on this day. You will still need to take in about 30 mg of iron daily to support the baby's growth.

*How I Feel* _____

_____

*My Thoughts* _____

_____

_____

# Day 257 Date _____

**Your baby on this day**

A whole network of cells was in place on this day, ready to begin forming your baby's digestive system, liver, and pancreas.

**Your body on this day**

You may have experienced some mild cramping at this point and an increase in the amount of vaginal discharge. Perhaps these symptoms tipped you off that you were pregnant.

*How I Feel* _____

_____

*My Thoughts* _____

_____

_____

# Day 256 Date _____

**Your baby on this day**

Today, a dedicated team of cells set out to form your baby's heart, blood vessels, muscles, and skeleton.

**Your body on this day**

Your body began to absorb more calcium from your food and was ready to draw from your own supply of calcium if necessary to support your baby's growth.

How I Feel _____

_____

My Thoughts _____

_____

## Day 255 Date_____

Your baby on this day

Your baby's body was looking more like a body. If you could have seen her, she would have resembled an upside down teardrop. The rounded top would be her head and the point of the teardrop would be her bottom.

Your body on this day

You may have felt unusually tired on this day, as your body was busy at work molding a little human being.

How I Feel _____

_____

My Thoughts _____

_____

## Day 254 Date _____

Your baby on this day

Today, cells grouped together along the center of your baby's body and formed a tunnel called the neural tube. On this day, your child had a very early brain and nervous system!

Your body on this day

By now you may have noticed a metallic taste in your mouth, a soreness in your breasts, fatigue or nausea. Some women don't notice any changes in their body in early pregnancy.

How I Feel _____

_____

My Thoughts _____

_____

## Day 253 Date _____

**Your baby on this day**

Today your baby's heart took shape! A group of cells moved into a U-formation in the area that has become your baby's chest. If a few weeks have passed since this day, his tiny little heart has already started beating.

**Your body on this day**

Your risk of a yeast infection increased when you became pregnant and your body started producing more estrogen. If at any point in your pregnancy you experience itching, irritation, unusual discharge or a burning sensation when urinating, tell your doctor so you can be treated right away.

How I Feel _____

_____

My Thoughts _____

_____

*Officially Pregnant!*

Gestational Week 3, LMP Week 5

## Day 252 Date _____

**Your baby today**

Your baby's blood vessel system is being born today, in a very primitive form. A system of cells is forming into tubes that will eventually transport blood throughout your baby's tiny body.

*For your baby*

Stay far away from cigarettes. Women who smoke during pregnancy are more likely to have a child with low birth weight and heart defects.

**Your body today**

If you're on a regular 28-day menstrual cycle and you don't get your period today, than you are officially "late"!

*For your body*

Many drugstore pregnancy tests can detect pregnancy (with great accuracy) from the first day of your missed period. Ready to find out? The best time to give yourself a urine test is first thing in the morning when your urine is most concentrated.

How I Feel _____

_____

My Thoughts _____

_____

**Your baby today**

Your baby is a collection of developing cells no bigger than a poppy seed. Your placenta is maturing into an incredible baby support system, readying itself to supply nutrients and oxygen to the baby for the rest of his or her time in your uterus.

**For your baby**

It's best to start taking prenatal vitamins as soon as you decide you want to conceive. If you haven't added prenatal vitamins to your daily routine yet, start today. To remind yourself to take them, place them at eye level or near your toothbrush—somewhere you know you'll see them every day.

**Your body today**

Women only have about a 20–30 percent chance of getting pregnant each month. Because of these odds, it can take couples up to a year or more to conceive. If you took a pregnancy test and it was positive, enjoy knowing that your body has achieved something rare and wonderful!

**For your body**

If you don't already have an OBGYN or midwife whom you know and trust, start asking around for recommendations. Don't be afraid to interview several medical professionals so you can choose the one with which you're most comfortable and confident.

> I opted for a doctor because I felt it was the safest way to go . . . if something went wrong during delivery or if there was something wrong with the baby, I felt the most comfortable with an M.D.
>
> —Maki, mother of 8-month-old Ha Min

How I Feel _____

_____

My Thoughts _____

_____

_____

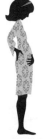

Week 3 Weigh-in:_____lbs

**Your baby today**

Your baby's head is beginning to grow fairly rapidly and will be disproportionately large for quite some time. Right now, she looks a little bit like a tadpole.

*For your baby*

You may be anxious to see the doctor, but most medical providers won't want to see you until eight weeks after your last menstrual period. Take care of yourself and wait it out.

**Your body today**

You probably haven't gained any weight yet, but you may be curious about what's to come. The usual amount of weight gain for pregnant women of normal weight is between 25–40 pounds, with most of that weight gain occurring near the end of pregnancy.

*For your body*

Take time to appreciate your figure in these first few weeks of pregnancy, because it will soon change considerably. Have someone take regular photos of your growing belly throughout this pregnancy so you can record your body's transformation as it unfolds.

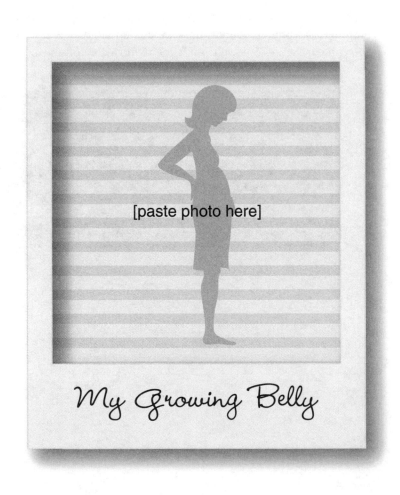

[paste photo here]

*My Growing Belly*

How I Feel _____

My Thoughts _____

# Day 249  Date_____

**Your baby today**

The upper portion of your baby's neural tube is beginning to develop into her brain.

**For your baby**

If you have a cat, use gloves when changing its litter box or have someone else do this chore for you. Contaminated cat feces can carry a disease called toxoplasmosis, which has been known to cause fetal death, pre-term labor, and birth defects.

**Your body today**

If you've experienced morning sickness already, then you may have discovered that its name is highly deceptive. It can strike at any time of day and it can last throughout the day. Roughly half of women experience some level of morning sickness during pregnancy.

**For your body**

There are many theories about how to alleviate nausea during pregnancy, but you may discover that few or none of them make the nausea disappear completely. Getting ample sleep and keeping a little bit of food (like dry crackers) in your stomach at all times are probably the most failsafe methods for managing this uncomfortable feeling.

How I Feel _____

My Thoughts _____

# Day 248  Date_____

**Your baby today**

Your little one's eyes and ears are beginning to make their debut today. You won't know your baby's true eye color until several months after she is born.

**For your baby**

Though there is no proof that dying your hair during pregnancy can cause harm to your baby, most doctors will advise you to hold off on that color change until after you deliver.

**Your body today**

Speaking of hair, you may have already noticed changes in your hair's thickness or shininess. Pregnancy hormones can alter the volume and texture of your hair.

*For your body*

If your hair gets thicker and shinier, enjoy the natural beauty boost. If your hair seems to be thinner and dryer, increase your iron and protein intake and give yourself a daily ten-minute scalp massage to counteract the problem.

*How I Feel* _____

_____

*My Thoughts* _____

_____

# Day 247 Date _____

Your baby today

Arm and leg buds are beginning to slowly emerge and your baby's skeleton is starting to form.

*For your baby*

Enjoy thinking about your baby today. You may even want to splurge on a onesie or a cute, gender-neutral outfit that you can hang somewhere prominent. Something as simple as this can make your pregnancy feel more real.

Your body today

Many women become stressed and fearful of miscarriage at this stage of pregnancy. You may even be concerned about how good a mother you will be.

*For your body*

Make it a point to share your worries with someone you love. While miscarriage can be a lingering concern in the first trimester, chances are you will continue to be pregnant and give birth to a healthy child. There's nothing wrong with assuming the best.

> I had several miscarriages before so I didn't fully believe I was pregnant until the first ultrasound. To see the tiny little life with that beating heart brought so much elation and relief that I finally began to enjoy being pregnant.
>
> —Cristina, mother of 2-year-old José

How I Feel _____

My Thoughts _____

## Day 246 Date _____

**Your baby today**

Your baby measures about .118 inches from crown to rump and has the beginnings of a yolk sac through which he'll receive precious nutrients.

**For your baby**

The amount of pesticides found on fruits and vegetables is not a significant health risk to a healthy adult, but a fetus is more vulnerable. You may want to switch to organic fruits and veggies while you're pregnant. If you're going to pick just a few organic fruits to splurge on, go with peaches, strawberries, and apples. The non-organic versions tend to carry high level of pesticides.

**Your body today**

Your breasts have already started to change and grow and will continue to do so. It's normal for a pregnant woman's breasts to go up two bra sizes during pregnancy.

**For your body**

Don't splurge on any new bras in your old size, since they probably won't fit for long. Save your money for later when you'll need bigger bras to keep up with your growing breasts.

How I Feel _____

My Thoughts _____

Gestational Week 4, LMP Week 6

## Day 245 Date _____

**Your baby today**

Your baby's heart is beating regularly today, pumping a miniscule amount of blood through an intricate new system of blood vessels.

**For your baby**

If you have any history of heart disease in your family or if the baby's father has history of heart disease, be sure to tell your doctor or midwife when you go to your first appointment. That way, she can be on the lookout for any problems with your baby's budding heart.

Week 4 Weigh-in: _____lbs

| Your body today | Your body is hungry for vitamins, but you may get sick to your stomach just thinking about swallowing those giant prenatal pills. |
|---|---|
| *For your body* | Don't avoid taking your prenatal vitamins, even if you are sick to your stomach or vomiting. Ask your doctor if there is a chewable version that you can take instead. |

How I Feel _____

_____

My Thoughts _____

_____

## Day 244 Date _____

| Your baby today | The separate portions of your child's brain are beginning to form and distinguish themselves. |
|---|---|
| *For your baby* | Avoid aspirin, ibuprofen and any other unnecessary medications during pregnancy. Aspirin and ibuprofen have both been linked to miscarriage and baby heart defects. Ibuprofen use in the third trimester is even riskier as it may lead to a dangerous decrease in the amount of amniotic fluid. If you need pain relief, stick with acetaminophen or speak with your doctor about other options. |
| Your body today | Hormonal changes may be slowing the movement of food through your digestive system. As a result, constipation can occur. |
| *For your body* | To ease constipation, make sure you eat foods high in fiber (like bran, fruits, and raw vegetables) while increasing your water intake. Exercise can also help to alleviate the problem. |

How I Feel _____

_____

My Thoughts _____

_____

## Day 243 Date _____

| Your baby today | Your baby's kidneys are evolving and will soon be able to produce tiny drops of urine. |
|---|---|

For your baby

While moderate amounts of caffeine (one or two cups of coffee a day) should not have a negative impact on your child, it's best to limit your caffeine intake from the very beginning of your pregnancy. Some studies cite a link between high amounts of caffeine during pregnancy and low birth weight in babies.

Your body today

A surge in your hormone levels plus an increase in your blood volume may lead to occasional headaches. Headaches are a common pregnancy symptom, especially in the first and third trimesters.

For your body

Try to alleviate headaches by relaxing in a dark room, taking a soothing bath, getting a massage, or applying a cold compress to the back of your neck. If that doesn't work, your medical provider may recommend that you take some acetaminophen to relieve the pain.

How I Feel _____

_____

My Thoughts _____

_____

_____

# Day 242 Date _____

Your baby today

Your baby's tiny arm and leg buds are becoming more pronounced. In just a few weeks, she will be able to move them all around.

For your baby

Avoid sleeping with an electric blanket during the first trimester of your pregnancy. Some studies have linked their use in early pregnancy to miscarriage and neural tube defects. While no one is sure whether these blankets are truly dangerous, the electric and magnetic fields (EMFs) they employ and their ability to significantly raise your core body temperature are enough of a threat to justify avoiding them.

Your body today

The beginning of pregnancy can be frustrating. One of the things you may wrestle with is when it's okay to tell family, friends, and coworkers that you're pregnant.

For your body

This may help ease your mind: Once your doctor has seen or heard evidence of a beating heart in your child, the chances that you'll miscarry are minimal. Some women still choose to make the announcement about 12 or 13 weeks from their last menstrual period (somewhere around Day 196 in this book), when the risk of miscarriage drops significantly. Others prefer to think positively and spread their good news freely.

How I Feel _____

_____

*My Thoughts* _____
_____
_____

# Day 241  Date _____

**Your baby today**    Slowly but surely, a nose and mouth are taking shape on your baby's face.

*For your baby*    Pick up a baby-naming book this week or cruise the Internet for baby-naming sites and star selecting a few favorites for each gender.

**Your body today**    Due to increased blood flow, you may be one of the lucky women who experience heightened sexual desire during this time. Some women, of course, feel just the opposite—especially i they are plagued by morning sickness.

*For your body*    Don't be afraid to enjoy sex with your partner at any time during your pregnancy. The onl things that should dissuade you from sex are: the advice of your medical provider, bleeding symptoms of a yeast or urinary tract infection, or general discomfort. Otherwise, enjoy no having to worry about birth control for a while!

*How I Feel* _____
_____

*My Thoughts* _____
_____

# Day 240  Date _____

**Your baby today**    Your baby's reproductive organs are just starting to form. The cells that will create eggs o sperm in your girl or boy are making their way to these organs.

*For your baby*    Finding out your baby's gender is just one of many ways to bond with your child while he o she is still in your womb. Some people prefer to leave this surprise for delivery day. Discus with your partner whether or not you should find out the gender ahead of time. Don't worr if you disagree—there is still plenty of time to resolve the issue.

**Your body today**    Certain physical conditions can add a level of risk to your pregnancy. If you are under ag 15 or over 35, have had pregnancy complications in the past, or are pregnant with multiples you are considered "high risk."

*For your body*    Don't let the classification of "high risk" concern you. While the label has a negative connotation it also means that you and your baby will benefit from extra care and attention.

My Thoughts

> There was a part of me that really wanted to know the gender, but I respected my husband's wish for a surprise and decided I could wait to find out. I'm sort of hoping it may make the labor just a bit easier because I'll be so excited to find out what I'm having!
>
> —Elena D., 6 months pregnant

## Day 239 Date _____

**Your baby today**

If you measured your baby's body today, it would be about a quarter of an inch long.

**For your baby**

It's still under debate whether eating peanuts or peanut products during pregnancy increases the chance that your baby will develop a peanut allergy. It's probably best to avoid peanuts for the next 238 days just to be safe. This is even more important if you or your baby's dad has a family history of peanut allergies.

**Your body today**

'Exhausted' may be the word that best describes your physical condition today. Getting through your work day during early pregnancy without falling asleep is a common challenge among pregnant women.

**For your body**

Steal some sleep whenever you can. Use your lunch break to catch a few z's in your car, tuck yourself into bed earlier at night, or shorten your morning routine so you can sleep in as late as possible. Remember, this will soon pass.

How I Feel

## Day 238 Date _____

**Your baby today**

Your baby's arm buds are lengthening and it's suddenly possible to distinguish the uppe portion from the lower portion. The shoulders are now discernable, too.

*For your baby*

Stay away from unpasteurized drinks and foods where bacteria like listeria can grow Pregnant women are twenty times more likely to become infected with listeria from food like soft cheeses, deli meats, or pâtés. Preterm labor and stillbirth could result.

**Your body today**

Instead of gaining weight, you may find that you are losing it because of morning sickness and/or food aversions.

*For your body*

Don't stress if you've lost a few pounds instead of gained. This is fairly normal and should stop as soon as your morning sickness subsides. If you find that you can't keep food down and are losing more and more weight, consult with your medical provider.

How I Feel _____

My Thoughts _____

## Day 237 Date _____

**Your baby today**

Your baby makes its first attempt at movement around this time. A slight shudder is about all he can manage right now, but just wait until you feel what he can do in a few months!

*For your baby*

Make sure you get at least 3 servings of fruits today. One apple, half a cup of orange juice and ¼ cup of raisins is all you and your baby need. For the American Pregnancy Association's complete nutritional guidelines, go to http://www.americanpregnancy.org/pregnancyhealth pregnancynutrition.html.

**Your body today**

You may be experiencing some intense food cravings today. The most common pregnancy food craving is fruit. Other common cravings include dairy products, chocolate, salty snacks and pickles.

*For your body*

Cravings are sometimes an indication of a food that's missing in your diet. Listen to you body and enjoy one of the greatest joys of pregnancy: permission to indulge your cravings!

How I Feel

My Thoughts

## Day 236 Date _____

**Your baby today**

Your baby's paddle-shaped hands are beginning to separate into fingers. Engraved on each paddle is the faint outline of five little digits.

**For your baby**

Start thinking about where you'll put the baby's room or crib. Your newborn will probably spend at least the first few weeks in your bedroom—more if you're a firm believer in co-sleeping—but it's still important to designate an area of the house just for him.

**Your body today**

Have you noticed that the skin around your nipple is turning darker in color? It's a surprising, but normal, pregnancy symptom.

**For your body**

The darkening of the areola is common during pregnancy. It may even be nature's way of guiding your baby to your milk sources once she's born. You'll find that your skin changes in many surprising ways in the coming months. The best thing you can do for your skin overall is to moisturize and drink lots of water. It will need to stretch quite a bit to accommodate your growing belly so lending it a little extra elasticity can only help

How I Feel

My Thoughts

## Day 235 Date _____

**Your baby today**

Your baby's eye color is slowly coming in today. Her eyes are always open at this point in her development. In a few weeks, they'll be shielded by brand new eyelids!

**For your baby**

Working should not pose a hazard to your unborn child, unless you have a very physically demanding job or one that exposes you to chemotherapy drugs, lead, or x-rays.

Week 5 Weigh-in:_____lbs

| Your body today | If you're feeling sick, hang in there. Most morning sickness resolves itself by the beginnin of the second trimester. If you're not feeling sick, it doesn't signify that something's wron with your pregnancy or your child. It just means that you're lucky. Kick back and enjoy. |
| For your body | If you are battling morning sickness, you may want to get into the habit of eating lots c small meals throughout the day. Having a little something in your stomach should help eas some of the nausea. |

How I Feel _____

My Thoughts _____

_____

# Day 234 Date _____

| Your baby today | In the last 48 hours, your baby's brain has developed by leaps and bounds and has becom 25 percent larger in size. Experts estimate that your baby's brain gains a quarter of a millio neurons (on average) every minute! |
| For your baby | A fever of over 103 degrees Fahrenheit can be very dangerous to your baby at this time, so b sure to let your doctor know if you spike a fever. Taking acetaminophen products or sitting i a tepid bath are some ways to keep your temperature down. |
| Your body today | If you're like many women, you'll feel nauseous today from the minute you wake up. |
| For your body | Don't be afraid to ask your doctor for anti-nausea medication. It does exist, and it works fc some people. In the meantime, leave some crackers by your bedside so you can nibble few before standing up and starting your day. |

How I Feel _____

_____

My Thoughts _____

_____

_____

# Day 233 Date _____

| Your baby today | Your baby has nostril openings now. Cells are gathering around the rims of those nostrils t build upon your baby's developing nose. |

While fish have plenty of nutritional benefits to offer your unborn child, the FDA advises pregnant women to avoid eating shark, swordfish, king mackerel and tilefish due to high levels of mercury. Albacore tuna can be eaten in limited portions (up to 6 ounces per week). The best thing you can do for your baby is to enjoy a variety of fish low in mercury such as shrimp, canned light tuna, salmon, pollock, and catfish.

**our body today**

You may feel like there is no end to the amount of saliva your mouth produces. Rest assured that it's not in your mind. And once again, those raging pregnancy hormones are to blame.

**or your body**

If the amount of excess saliva is bothering you or aggravating your morning sickness, you may want to try drinking more water or sucking on hard candies. If that doesn't work, brushing your teeth a few extra times a day may make you feel a little better.

How I Feel

My Thoughts

# Day 232 Date _____

**our baby today**

Your baby's legs have now lengthened to look less like buds and more like legs. The outline of a thigh, calf, and foot can already be seen.

**or your baby**

Make a dentist appointment today to ensure that your teeth and gums are healthy. Gum swelling and gum disease are more common during pregnancy (due to those crazy hormones) and may actually be linked to preterm labor. Practice good oral hygiene and be sure to let your dentist know that you are pregnant when you show up for your next appointment.

**our body today**

You may be enduring some strange first-trimester symptoms like a metallic taste in your mouth, extra burping and farting, or a stuffy nose.

**or your body**

If you have any of these symptoms, rest assured that you're suffering through them along with many other pregnant women. Try to adopt a new, lighthearted attitude about these things knowing that they won't last. Easier said than done, right?

How I Feel

My Thoughts

# Day 231 Date _____

### Your baby today

Your baby's mouth has lips and the beginnings of a tongue today!

### For your baby

Look into cord blood banking today and decide whether it's for you. You don't have to mak any decisions now, but it doesn't hurt to know the facts ahead of time. Some parents pa to have private companies store their baby's umbilical cord blood as a sort of insurance i case their child gets a serious pediatric disorder. The blood can be used in transplant to trea disorders like sickle cell disease and leukemia. It's free to donate your baby's cord blood t a public cord bank, but it doesn't offer the same health guarantees for your child.

### Your body today

Your fatigue and food aversions may be at their peak today. One whiff of an unappetizin food and you may find yourself bolting to the bathroom.

### For your body

Let your instincts guide you today and every day. Your fatigue and your likely tendency t avoid more "adventurous" foods during this time may be a natural safeguard against th many foreign substances that can harm your developing child.

How I Feel _____

_____

_____

My Thoughts _____

_____

_____

# Day 230 Date _____

### Your baby today

Your baby now has an upper and lower jaw.

### For your baby

Don't take chances by eating leftovers that have been sitting in your fridge for more than few days or food that seems a little on the raw side. Now is the time to play it safe.

### Your body today

You may already be tired of having to think twice about everything you eat. The guy at th deli counter may roll his eyes at you today when you ask whether that tuna salad is mad with albacore or light tuna.

### For your body

Cutting back on food and drinks you used to enjoy and being more particular about wha you eat is a burden, but you may find that it gets easier with time. One way to make you pregnancy diet more bearable is to find new indulgences. With creative "mocktails" t replace your alcoholic drink of choice and mouthwatering snacks that combine your late food cravings, you might just enjoy the next 229 days.

How I Feel _____

My Thoughts _____

> Before I was pregnant, I assumed alcohol would be the toughest thing to give up. Ironically, it was not as bad as I thought because I didn't crave alcohol at all when I was pregnant. I don't know if it was a physical or psychological aversion or what. Every once in a while I would have a small glass of wine or beer, but never more than one drink.
>
> —Carolyn S., mother of 1-year-old Simon

## Day 229 Date _____

**Your baby today**

Tiny tooth buds now line the inside of your baby's mouth. They are the beginnings of her primary (baby) teeth. You may not see the actual baby teeth emerge until she's about six months old.

**For your baby**

Check your employee manual today to see if you are eligible for any paid maternity leave. You may get as much as twelve weeks of unpaid leave to care for your baby if you meet the guidelines of the Family and Medical Leave Act. Go to http://www.dol.gov/esa/whd/fmla/ for more information.

**Your body today**

Your friends and coworkers may be starting to notice that growing bulge at your middle. You will probably feel a little bloated and uncomfortable in your normal pants and jeans.

**For your body**

If you're not ready to invest in maternity clothes just yet, stick with elastic waist skirts and dresses that allow a little extra room for the baby bump. Maternity clothing stores and online retailers offer several kinds of stretchy bands that can be worn to hold up—and conceal the waistline of—your unbuttoned or unzipped pants.

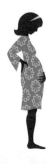

Week 6 Weigh-in: _____lbs

How I Feel _____

My Thoughts _____

## Day 228 Date _____

**Your baby today**

Your baby just gained the ability to cry. Tear ducts have started to form in the corner of both eyes. One day, those tears will move you to do just about anything!

*For your baby*

This is the week when most women head to their OB/GYN or midwife to confirm the pregnancy and make sure the baby is in good health. Early prenatal care is crucial to the ongoing health of your baby, so make an appointment today if you haven't already.

**Your body today**

Soon you may get a glimpse inside your own body to see that little baby growing inside you. If your prenatal appointment is today, get ready to start bonding with that little being. Once you see his little flickering heart on the screen, you'll be absolutely amazed and probably a little reassured. Your chance of miscarriage goes way down once you see or hear a heartbeat in your baby. You'll also get a better idea of how far along you are: In the first half of pregnancy, ultrasound is able to predict your baby's age fairly accurately, give or take about a week.

*For your body*

In addition to an ultrasound, your first prenatal visit will probably include a review of your health and family health history, a physical exam, pap smear, cervical screening, and due date prediction. Write down any questions you have before you go so you don't forget anything.

How I Feel _____

My Thoughts _____

**our baby today**  Your family's ears (or your partner's family's ears) have already been passed down to your baby. At this point, his ears reveal all the unique characteristics determined by his genetics.

**or your baby**  If possible, invite your baby's father to become more involved in your pregnancy. Whether it's attending prenatal appointments, reading a book about your baby's growth, or writing a few entries in this journal, present some practical ways that he can play a role. Don't be disappointed if he doesn't seem to think about the baby non-stop. Chalk it up to the fact that his body is not the center of the action.

**our body today**  You may miss working out or exercising as much as you used to before you were nauseous and tired all the time.

**or your body**  If you love working out and/or running, you don't have to stop just because you're pregnant. You can continue to do so well into your pregnancy as long as you clear it with your doctor. Doing so may even help some of that former energy return.

How I Feel _____

_____

_____

My Thoughts _____

_____

_____

_____

**our baby today**  Your baby's fingers are longer now and look more like fingers. Soon her one-of-a-kind fingerprints will be permanently etched on all ten tips.

**or your baby**  Don't be afraid to eat fat when you're pregnant. Avoid processed fats and pre-packaged foods in favor of the healthy fats you get from fish, nuts, avocados, and vegetable oils. Healthy fats like these help build your baby's brain and nervous system.

**our body today**  You may have noticed that your breasts have gotten noticeably larger in the last month. Your partner may have noticed as well. Prepare yourself for them to get even bigger in the second trimester and to change shape after pregnancy.

*For your body*

Wearing a supportive bra day and night throughout pregnancy may not be the mos comfortable option, but it could prevent some of the sagging that naturally occurs as a resu of pregnancy.

*How I Feel* _____

_____

_____

*My Thoughts* _____

_____

_____

## Day 225 Date _____

**Your baby today**

If you could see a profile shot of your baby, you'd get your first glimpse of the tip of his nos What you might not see are the two separate air passages that have formed behind eac nostril. In just 224 days, your baby will take his first breath of air.

*For your baby*

Add some chickpeas to your salad today. Just one cup has 5 mg of iron to help boost you baby's red blood cell supply.

**Your body today**

Extreme morning sickness, a bulging belly and breasts, and/or a hard-to-contain level o excitement may make it difficult to keep your pregnancy a secret from anyone.

*For your body*

While many women wait until 12 to 14 weeks (LMP) to break the news at their workplac you may feel more than ready to let the word out. If you have a strong relationship wit your boss and coworkers or if your early pregnancy symptoms are interfering with your jo it might be a good idea to let them know you're pregnant. You may need the extra suppo that they can provide.

*How I Feel* _____

_____

*My Thoughts* _____

_____

_____

## Day 224 Date _____

**Your baby today**

Your baby is just over an inch long and about the size of a bean today. You can now official refer to him as your "little peanut," as he weighs about as much. Even with an ultrasound, would be difficult to discern the external genitals and determine the gender.

*or your baby*

You may want to start getting used to sleeping on your side during pregnancy. Sleeping on your stomach will soon be physically uncomfortable and, later in the pregnancy, so will sleeping on your back. Try sleeping on your left side tonight, as that position allows more blood to flow to your baby.

*our body today*

Your expanding uterus is pushing up against your bladder and making you have to pee more often. This sensation may hit you in the middle of the night when all you want to do is sleep.

*or your body*

There's nothing you can do to avoid this little nuisance completely, but you can prolong the urge to pee if you squeeze out all the urine in your bladder every time you go. Avoid beverages and foods that cause frequent urination like caffeinated drinks, cranberry juice, and asparagus.

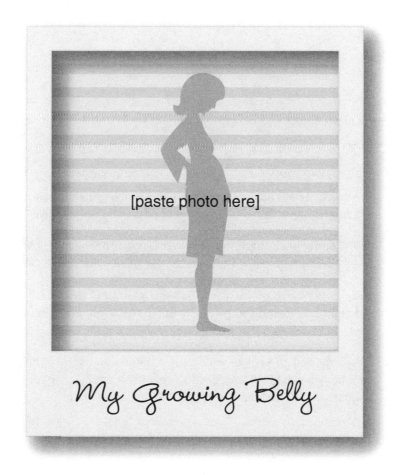

[paste photo here]

*My Growing Belly*

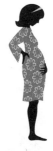

Week 7 Weigh-in:_____lbs

—Ria P., mother of 2-month-old Daniel

How I Feel _____

_____

My Thoughts _____

_____

_____

# Day 223 Date _____

| | |
|---|---|
| Your baby today | By now, your baby has lost some of his amphibious qualities and is looking much more human. His fingers are no longer entirely webbed and his tadpole-like "tail" has disappeared. |
| *For your baby* | If you don't get enough zinc early in pregnancy (15 mg a day), your baby could be at higher risk of preterm delivery. The best sources of zinc are whole grains, wheat germ, eggs, fish, meat, poultry, and yes, popcorn. |
| Your body today | Don't be surprised if you feel extra emotional these days and prone to fits of tears. This is just a normal part of early pregnancy. |
| *For your body* | Allow yourself to vent to your closest friends and your partner on days where you feel emotionally volatile. If you sense a "weepfest" coming on at the wrong time or place, quickly excuse yourself and make a beeline for the ladies' room. |

How I Feel _____

My Thoughts _____

_____

**Your baby today**
Your baby now has the foundation for every organ and bone it will need as a full-grown adult. Already, your baby can contract his or her muscles.

**For your baby**
Fill up on manganese today in the form of fruits, peas, whole grains, beans, nuts, tea, or cloves. It does wonders for organ development and your baby's hearing.

**Your body today**
You may experience mild to severe heartburn today after eating. Progesterone and estrogen have begun to soften the muscles and valves of your digestive tract, slowing the movement of food through your system.

**For your body**
Stop heartburn before it becomes an issue by eating small meals all day long instead of three big meals. Don't lie down after eating and stay away from spicy or greasy foods (unless, of course, satisfying the craving is worth it to you!).

How I Feel _____

_____

My Thoughts _____

_____

**Your baby today**
Today your baby's back is much straighter and his neck is starting to take shape. He can also make a fist now, and may figure out how to suck his own thumb!

**For your baby**
If you are over 35 years old or have a family history that warrants concern, you may want to talk to your doctor about chorionic villus sampling (CVS). You can have this diagnostic test done between weeks 10 and 12 (LMP) to detect chromosomal abnormalities like Down Syndrome and genetic disorders like cystic fibrosis with 98–99 percent accuracy.

**Your body today**
You have probably gained between 2 and 5 pounds in this first trimester of pregnancy. If you have gained a lot more, it may be time to re-evaluate your eating habits.

**For your body**
While you may have started doubling your portions in the spirit of "eating for two," all you really need to support your growing baby in the first trimester is about 100 extra calories per day. That equates to one healthy snack, like a half cup of 2 percent cottage cheese or a piece of fruit. In the second and third trimester, you'll need more like 300 additional calories per day. You can get about that many calories with a mini-meal of one scrambled egg and a slice of jelly wheat toast.

How I Feel _____

My Thoughts _____

## Day 220 Date _____

**Your baby today**

Your baby has just developed his own unique food preferences. His tongue is now covered in taste buds. One day, he will let you know loud and clear which foods he likes and which he doesn't.

*For your baby*

You and your partner may want to begin discussing what will happen after this baby is born. Will your child need daycare? Will you try to breastfeed? What are your expectations of each other once the baby is born? The earlier you smooth out these details, the less stress you'll have during pregnancy. The less stress you have during pregnancy, the happier your baby will be.

**Your body today**

You may experience a heightened sense of smell while you're pregnant. If you're feeling well enough, you might enjoy this new "super power," but if certain smells send waves of nausea through your body, you probably will not.

*For your body*

If you're dining out and become nauseated by a certain odor, ask for a glass of water with lemon. Sniffing and tasting lemon can help make you feel better immediately.

How I Feel _____

_____

_____

My Thoughts _____

_____

## Day 219 Date _____

**Your baby today**

Your baby's joints are working now so he is probably enjoying the novelty of bending his knees, elbows, shoulders, ankles, and wrists and moving freely about the amniotic sac.

*For your baby*

While herbal teas can be a perfectly acceptable and relaxing indulgence, avoid drinking them in excess as little is known about how herbs affect pregnancy. For a list of safe and unsafe teas and ingredients, go to http://www.americanpregnancy.org/pregnancyhealth/herbaltea.htm

**Your body today**

Don't panic if you blow your nose today and see a little bit of blood. Your hormones soften the lining of your nasal passages, which can lead to some bleeding. As your pregnancy progresses, occasional nosebleeds may be a fact of life.

**For your body**

Using a humidifier in your bedroom, drinking lots of fluids, and getting loads of vitamin C can all help to alleviate nosebleeds in pregnancy.

How I Feel _____

My Thoughts _____

_____

_____

# Day 218  Date _____

**Your baby today**

Your baby's heart is now a four-chambered organ featuring tiny valves. His or her body is as small as a grape, just about 1½ inches long.

**For your baby**

More and more women are turning to midwives and doulas to help them through their pregnancy and delivery. These specialists can be a great match for, among others, those who want to give birth with minimal medical intervention. You may want to do some research and decide whether either of these professionals is right for you.

**Your body today**

Increased blood flow to the area around the vagina combined with an increase in mucus production during pregnancy often leads to more vaginal discharge. If you notice that you have more discharge, rest assured that it's normal.

**For your body**

There isn't much you can do to avoid an increase in vaginal discharge, but you can stave off bacterial infections. Avoid tight pants, wear cotton underwear, and don't allow anything scented (like soap or bubble bath) to come near your vagina.

How I Feel _____

My Thoughts _____

_____

_____

# Day 217    Date _____

**Your baby today**

Today medical professionals no longer consider your baby just another embryo. She has earned the classification of fetus, meaning "offspring" in Latin, because all of the working parts of her body exist in their rightful place.

*For your baby*

Nutrition is of key importance throughout your pregnancy. In the first trimester, getting at least 400 mcg of folic acid per day can reduce the risk of neural tube defects—like spina bifida—by up to 75 percent.

**Your body today**

You may find that the strength of your fingernails has changed. They will either grow faster and stronger or will break more easily.

*For your body*

Eat lots of calcium-rich foods today if you need to rescue your fingernails from a brittle state. If you already consume a lot of calcium and aren't seeing the benefits, it may be that drinking lots of coffee, eating sugary foods, or feeling stressed is preventing you from absorbing the calcium you need.

How I Feel _____
_____
_____

My Thoughts _____
_____
_____
_____

# Day 216    Date _____

**Your baby today**

Your baby's heart assumes its final shape today and beats at about 140 beats per minute.

*For your baby*

Your doctor will use a special stethoscope or a hand-held Doppler ultrasound device to check your baby's heart rate at each prenatal visit. He or she will make sure that the fetal heart rate falls somewhere between 110 and 160 beats a minute (almost twice as fast as your own). An unchanging fetal heart rate or one that's too low or too high may indicate a problem.

**Your body today**

Was that a new pimple in the mirror this morning? Pregnancy can be kind to some women's skin, lending them a healthy glow, and cruel to others.

*For your body*

If acne outbreaks are troubling you, cut down on the amount of fat you eat, drink more water and exercise more often. Avoid using over-the-counter face creams to deal with the problem—chemicals in some face and acne creams could have a negative effect on your baby.

# Day 215   Date _____

**Your baby today**

Because of her rapid brain growth, your baby's head is still rather big in comparison to the rest of her body. There is a bulge at the front of her head that gives the brain extra room to grow.

**For your baby**

You will probably visit the OB/GYN or midwife about once a month during this part of your pregnancy. Sometime after 28 weeks (LMP), you'll see your doctor every two weeks. Once you hit Week 36, you will probably be scheduled for weekly visits.

> Midwives stay in the room with women throughout most of their labor, supporting them and guiding them—helping them push and then delivering the baby. This is a very important aspect of midwifery because studies have shown that a constant, calm presence in the labor room increases the rate of natural childbirth and decreases the rate of vacuum deliveries and C-sections.
>
> —Julie, Certified Nurse-Midwife

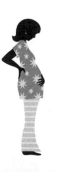

Week 8 Weigh-in:_____lbs

## Your body today

Your blood pressure is lower than usual today. It tends to decline during the first half of pregnancy and then returns to normal later on.

## For your body

A nurse or doctor will take your blood pressure reading every time you visit. While 120/70 is a normal reading, anything over 140/90 is a warning flag for high blood pressure. A pattern of rising blood pressure could indicate a serious condition called preeclampsia, which is also known as toxemia and is characterized by high blood pressure and fluid retention.

How I Feel _____

_____

My Thoughts _____

_____

# Day 214   Date _____

## Your baby today

Your baby's eyelids now cover her eyes and are fused shut. They will open around Week 2 (LMP) for the first time.

## For your baby

It may seem early to be thinking of child care, but if you are considering going back to work after your maternity leave then it's never too early. Popular daycare facilities can have long waiting lists, so don't cause your self unnecessary headaches by putting off the search until the end of your pregnancy or after your baby is born.

## Your body today

You may have "popped" by now, meaning your lower belly is gently rounded and you are more noticeably pregnant.

## For your body

Don't be surprised if you find yourself touching your stomach more often as you become increasingly aware of your baby's presence there. When your child gets big enough to feel them, she may find these stomach touches and massages very soothing.

How I Feel _____

_____

My Thoughts _____

_____

# Day 213   Date _____

## Your baby today

Your baby's feet are each about 1/10 of an inch long and are now actively kicking.

**For your baby**

You have been a trouper for your little baby for the last 53 days of your pregnancy. The very beginning and the very end of pregnancy are known for being the most difficult, so take pride in knowing that you've powered through a physically and emotionally trying period and have done lots of wonderful things for your growing child along the way. Keep up the good work!

**Your body today**

If you wear contact lenses, you may find that they are unusually dry and uncomfortable today.

**For your body**

Pregnancy dries out your eyes, so you may need to add rewetting drops throughout the day. If your lenses are still uncomfortable, it may be time to wear your glasses again.

How I Feel

My Thoughts

## Day 212    Date

**Your baby today**

Your baby's fingernails, toenails, and hair are starting to come in today.

**For your baby**

Hang in there, as you are only 23 days away from carrying your child through the first trimester. Once you hit the second trimester, your baby will have made it past the riskiest stage of his development.

**Your body today**

You may be having a hard time finding a suitable lunch replacement during pregnancy now that deli meats and hot dogs are deemed questionable (pregnant women are about 20 times more likely than the average adult to be infected by listeria from eating cured meats).

**For your body**

Don't despair if lunch meats are a staple in your diet. Switch to lunchtime salads and hot meals. If you're really craving that hot dog or that turkey sandwich, make sure that you reheat it until it's piping hot. As long as the meat is cooked well enough, it should be safe to eat.

How I Feel

My Thoughts

**Your baby today**

Your baby is just over 2 inches long, about the size of a lime. She weighs only a quarter of an ounce. Her weekly weight is now beginning to change more significantly.

*For your baby*

Douching when you're not pregnant is bad enough—it increases your chance of having a vaginal infection—but douching when you are pregnant is even worse. It's associated with preterm labor and low birth-weight babies.

**Your body today**

Have you noticed that your breasts look a little different today? More blood than usual is pumping to them to help them grow an extra layer of fat and extra milk glands. Because of this, you may notice a web of blue veins appearing over each breast.

*For your body*

Now's the time to shop for a new bra, one that will offer more support for those sensitive aching breasts. The blue lines may not go away for a while, but at least you will be more comfortable.

*How I Feel* _____

_____

*My Thoughts* _____

_____

_____

_____

> I found the comforting part of pregnancy was the understanding smiles I received from every pregnant woman and mom I passed. It felt like I was being inducted into a new sorority.
>
> —Antonia F., mother of 20-month-old Carmine

# Day 210  Date _____

**Your baby today**

Your baby can wiggle his tiny little toes now that they're separated.

**For your baby**

Soaking in water over 100 degrees could raise your baby's risk of neural tube defects and increase the chance of miscarriage. Steaming hot baths, saunas and hot tubs are best enjoyed once your little one is out of your body. If you're not sure of the water temperature, play it safe: get out before your skin becomes red or you begin to sweat.

**Your body today**

Your rib cage is widening and you may start breathing faster than usual. Eventually, you may experience some shortness of breath; as the baby takes up more room in your body, your lungs won't have as much room to expand.

**For your body**

If you have asthma or any other lung disorder, there's no need to be overly concerned. Most women with asthma are able to safely manage their breathing issues using the inhalers and medicines they normally use. Just make sure that your doctor is aware of your condition and has given you the green light to continue using your regular meds.

How I Feel _____

_____

My Thoughts _____

_____

# Day 209  Date _____

**Your baby today**

Your baby's bones are harder and stronger now. His skin, on the other hand, is so thin and transparent that it's possible to see the bones beneath.

**For your baby**

If you opt for a first trimester screening, which consists of a special blood test and ultrasound, your doctor can estimate your odds of carrying a child with Down syndrome or Edwards syndrome. If the odds are high enough to concern you, you can undergo further testing—though it may be more invasive and may pose some risk to your growing baby. When making a decision about prenatal tests and screening, always measure the risks against the value of knowing the results.

**Your body today**

Strange as it may sound, you may not be the only one in your household experiencing this pregnancy. Occasionally, something called Couvade syndrome causes sympathetic pregnancy symptoms in fathers. They put on weight, get nauseous and tired, and may even experience stomach cramps when you're in labor.

Week 9 Weigh-in: _____lbs

**For your body**    If your partner is experiencing symptoms of pregnancy, you may either be touched that he's in tune with your body or irritated by the notion that he's faking or competing for attention. Couvade has been scientifically researched and proven, so do your best to bear with him through this strange time in both your lives.

*How I Feel* _____

_____

*My Thoughts* _____

_____

_____

# Day 208 Date _____

**Your baby today**    Your baby's external genitals have almost finished forming. In about seven more weeks, an ultrasound technician could reveal whether you will give birth to a son or a daughter.

**For your baby**    If you don't know any lullabies or soothing songs by heart, today may be a good day to print out lyrics for (and memorize) a few favorites. Even in the womb, your baby is soothed by your voice. Imagine how comforting your singing will be when he makes the adjustment from the peaceful womb to the hectic, outside world.

**Your body today**    If you're like most pregnant women, you'll crave chocolate, ice cream, fruit, or salty chips today. If you have a condition called pica, you will instead crave non-food items like ice, clay, chalk, sand, or coal. This condition is unusual and is caused by the hormonal changes in your body.

**For your body**    It's best not to act on any extreme cravings during pregnancy. These urges may be a sign that you're lacking certain nutrients like iron and zinc. Let your medical provider know immediately.

*How I Feel* _____

_____

*My Thoughts* _____

_____

# Day 207 Date _____

**Your baby today**    Your baby's movements are becoming more and more varied. He may press his hands softly against his mouth or make fists and hold them up in front like a boxer.

**For your baby**

You may have enjoyed sushi before you were pregnant but now that you're looking out for someone else, raw fish is off limits. Raw fish can be a breeding ground for parasites and/or listeria bacteria. If you can't wait 29 more weeks, limit yourself to vegetarian or cooked sushi options.

**Your body today**

You're finding it hard to stay awake at work or at home, but you can't rely on coffee to fix the problem anymore. What's a pregnant girl to do?

**For your body**

Try getting up and stretching your arms and legs. Go for a brisk walk to get your blood flowing again. If you're still exhausted, arrange to go to bed extra-early tonight so you won't have the same problem tomorrow. Better yet, take a catnap when fatigue strikes if at all possible.

How I Feel

My Thoughts

# Day 206 Date _____

**Your baby today**

Your baby is already acting like a newborn. If you could peek inside your uterus today, you might see him swallowing, yawning, or sucking his finger.

**For your baby**

Calcium intake is crucial when it comes to giving your baby strong bones and teeth. Snacking on dairy products like cheese and yogurt and drinking lots of milk are the best ways to load up on calcium. To give you an idea of how much you need per day, three cups of milk or yogurt can satisfy your daily requirement.

**Your body today**

Your body, especially that slowly emerging bump in front, is like a magnet for eyes and hands. You may feel suddenly self-conscious about the attention or you may thoroughly enjoy it.

**For your body**

Time to get adjusted to the extra attention you will get throughout your entire pregnancy. For better or for worse, as soon as you start showing you become a walking fertility symbol and the recipient of many unsolicited belly rubs. Let people know if they cross the line and invade your personal space. Otherwise, try to enjoy the attention and let it remind you of how unique and amazing it is to be pregnant.

How I Feel

My Thoughts

# Day 205 Date _____

| | |
|---|---|
| Your baby today | Your baby's intestines are so long that they needed to develop outside of his body, extending into the umbilical cord. Today, those intestines have found their appropriate place inside his body. |
| *For your baby* | Wash all of your fruits and vegetables carefully before eating them, even the kind that say "pre-washed." Also make a habit of washing your hands more often to avoid picking up infections that could harm the baby. |
| Your body today | Your morning sickness may still be in full force. If you find yourself vomiting a lot today, your body may be losing precious stores of potassium. |
| *For your body* | Nothing is worse than being stuck in traffic, except maybe being stuck in traffic when you're pregnant and really hungry or sick to your stomach. Keep bland foods like a sleeve of crackers or a bag of almonds in your car for quick energy and to help keep nausea at bay. If vomiting is an issue for you, snack on a banana or two (if you can keep it down) during the course of the day to help restore some of that lost potassium. |

How I Feel _____

_____

My Thoughts _____

_____

# Day 204 Date _____

| | |
|---|---|
| Your baby today | Your baby is over 2½ inches long from crown to rump and weighs about half an ounce. |
| *For your baby* | If you're traveling by air anytime soon, you may be unsure whether the security x-ray machines are a danger to your baby. It's not known for sure whether the low levels of nonionizing radiation (safer than the ionizing radiation performed in hospitals) can do any harm to your baby. If you are concerned or if you travel frequently, you may want to opt for a personal search by a security agent. |
| Your body today | Your pelvic-floor muscles may already be more relaxed than before pregnancy, causing you to leak a little urine when you laugh or sneeze. |
| *For your body* | Doing a few minutes of Kegel exercises each day can help strengthen those pelvic floor muscles and help you avoid embarrassing leaks. Squeeze the muscle you use to stop your urine flow, hold, and release. As an added bonus, Kegels can help empower you to push more effectively during labor. |

*How I Feel* _____

_____

*My Thoughts* _____

_____

_____

# Day 203 Date _____

**Your baby today**  Your baby is experiencing bouts of hiccups today, even if you are not yet aware of them. These hiccups may help to exercise her diaphragm in preparation for the work it will do when breathing oxygen.

**For your baby**  Get some fluoride to your baby in the form of an apple and a few glasses of tap water (check your town Web site to see if your tap water is fortified with fluoride). You'll be helping your little boy or girl build a mouthful of healthy teeth.

**Your body today**  Your uterus is so enlarged that your doctor can feel it by pressing on your lower abdomen.

**For your body**  Keep up your energy level by engaging in a sport you enjoy like running, yoga, bicycling, or swimming. If you're concerned that you're working your body too hard, get a watch that tracks your heart rate and keep it under 140 beats per minute.

*How I Feel* _____

_____

*My Thoughts* _____

_____

_____

# Day 202 Date _____

**Your baby today**  Your baby is now starting to show off his facial features, some of which are similar to your own. He looks different from other babies her age already, from the shape of his eyes and ears to the finer contours of his face.

**For your baby**  You may have an image in your mind of what your child will look like, but be prepared for a surprise. Thanks to the twists and turns of heredity, he may inherit some surprising qualities buried deep in your genetics—like your great-grandmother's red hair!

Week 10 Weigh-in: _____ lbs

| Your body today | Today you may notice small, dark splotches on your face or neck. These are called chloasma or the "mask" of pregnancy. |
| --- | --- |
| For your body | Hang in there. These dark patches almost always go away after you deliver your baby. In the meantime, some concealer and/or foundation may make them less noticeable. |

How I Feel _____

_____

_____

My Thoughts _____

_____

_____

# Day 201  Date _____

| Your baby today | Your baby just got her voice! Her vocal cords are now forming and will continue to do so until the day she lets out her first cry—to the delight of everyone in the delivery room. |
| --- | --- |
| For your baby | Sixty grams of protein per day helps support your baby's tissue growth. Chicken, eggs, fish, nuts, and beans are all great sources of protein. Aim for three servings of a combination of protein sources every day, like a hard-boiled egg with breakfast and a chicken-and-bean burrito for lunch. |
| Your body today | You may find yourself holding on tighter to railings and watching your step more carefully due to fear of falling while pregnant. |
| For your body | Contrary to what you see in the movies, taking a fall at this early stage of pregnancy will probably not lead to miscarriage. The uterus is still so low in your pelvis and protected by your pelvic bones that it's unlikely any harm would be done. That said, you may want to cancel those future skiing or horseback riding plans since a serious fall in your 2nd or 3rd trimester could be highly dangerous. |

How I Feel _____

_____

_____

My Thoughts _____

_____

_____

# Day 200 Date _____

**Your baby today**

Your baby's pituitary gland, located at the base of her brain, is now sophisticated enough to emit hormones that regulate growth, metabolism, and blood pressure.

**For your baby**

Eat foods with lots of omega-3 fatty acids (salmon is a great source). Omega-3s are good for your little one's brain and visual development.

**Your body today**

Early pregnancy can be extremely exciting, but it can also be stressful when you're trying to cope with morning sickness while maintaining your usual busy lifestyle. Allow yourself to let things slide a bit as you fight through these last few weeks of morning sickness. Chances are, you'll feel better soon and can catch up when you do.

**For your body**

Omega-3 foods aren't just for developing babies. You can also benefit from eating omega-3 rich foods like walnuts and cold-water fish, as they can ward off high blood pressure during pregnancy.

How I Feel _____

_____

My Thoughts _____

_____

_____

# Day 199 Date _____

**Your baby today**

Your baby's digestive system has developed by leaps and bounds. By today it can absorb glucose and sugar and make the contractions that push food through the bowels.

**For your baby**

Now is a good time to work up a new budget reflecting the added costs of having a baby. Hospital and doctor bills, diapers, formula, and clothes can quickly add up. If you're not sure where to start, try this baby cost calculator from BabyCenter.com to figure out approximately how much money you'll need in the first year: http://www.babycenter.com/babyCostCalculator.htm.

**Your body today**

Your skin may start to itch from all the stretching it's doing, especially if you're gaining weight fast. If stretch marks run in your family, you may start to see signs of them soon.

**For your body**

Don't be suckered into buying expensive creams that promise to prevent stretch marks from forming. There's no proof that any of them can actually live up to this promise. Moisturize to treat dryness and itchiness. If you want to give your skin more elasticity, eat foods rich in protein and vitamin C.

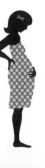

# Day 198   Date _____

**Your baby today**   Today your baby is practicing jumping by rebounding off your uterine wall. She is opening and closing her arms and twisting and turning her whole body in what are surprisingly graceful movements.

*For your baby*   Grab a healthy snack like apple slices lightly coated in melted cheddar cheese. Fiber and calcium are a great team in terms of taste and nutritional value for your baby.

**Your body today**   This is an awkward phase for many women. You're showing, but not so much that everyone assumes the extra weight is pregnancy related. You may either be unbelievably proud of your growing breasts and belly or increasingly self-conscious.

*For your body*   Joining a prenatal yoga class is a great way to stay connected to your new body as it changes. It can increase your strength and flexibility, make you feel better about yourself, and help introduce you to other expecting moms in your area.

*How I Feel* _____

_____

*My Thoughts* _____

_____

# Day 197   Date _____

**Your baby today**   When you cough, laugh, sneeze, or walk, your baby rocks gently back and forth in the resulting amniotic waves.

*For your baby*   No need to muffle a sneeze on account of your baby. She will get used to all of your movements and is even comforted by your physical activity and sounds.

**Your body today**   Most of the weight you are gaining now is baby weight, but a substantial portion also reflects maternal fat and nutrient stores as well as extra fluids that build up during pregnancy.

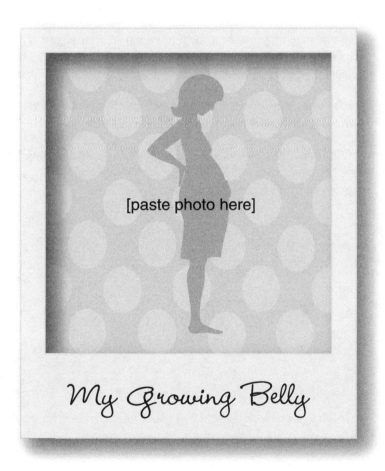

[paste photo here]

*My Growing Belly*

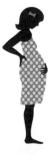

| For your body | Slow and steady wins the race when it comes to gaining weight during pregnancy. If you can avoid putting on a lot of weight all at once, you may also avoid having hemorrhoids, varicose veins, stretch marks, backache, fatigue, indigestion, and shortness of breath during your pregnancy. |

How I Feel _____

My Thoughts _____
_____
_____

## Day 196 Date _____

| Your baby today | Your baby is about 3 inches long from the top of her head to her rump. When you push down on certain areas of your belly, your baby may respond by squirming. |

| For your baby | Sprinkle some granola or a favorite cereal in your yogurt today for a healthy combo of calcium, protein, and fiber. The calcium will help build baby's bones and teeth, the protein helps her produce new cells, and the fiber rids your body of extra fat and cholesterol. |

| Your body today | If your breasts feel lumpier than usual today, it's because your milk ducts are growing and stretching to hold the milk you'll need for your baby. |

| For your body | Continue with regular breast self-exams as if you weren't pregnant. If you're having a hard time knowing which lumps are pregnancy related and which are cause for concern, let an expert (a doctor or specialist) decide. |

How I Feel _____
_____

My Thoughts _____
_____
_____

## Day 195 Date _____

| Your baby today | Your baby has new reflexes! If you could rub his palms, he would close his fingers around yours. If you could rub the bottom of his feet, his toes would curl. |

| For your baby | Vomiting and fever is the last thing you and your baby need. If it's flu season and you haven't already received the flu vaccine, make arrangements to do so. |

**our body today**

Suddenly your contact lenses or glasses are failing you. That's because pregnancy hormones have initiated changes in your vision (usually for the worse) that can temporarily alter your prescription.

**or your body**

It's safe to get an eye exam during pregnancy, but it might not be worth the trouble. If you're like most women, your eyesight is only slightly different and will return to normal after you deliver the baby. Severely blurred vision, on the other hand, can be a sign of gestational diabetes or high blood pressure and should be brought to a doctor's attention.

How I Feel

My Thoughts

## Day 194    Date _____

**our baby today**

Your baby's body is beginning to get a soft layer of hair called lanugo. This hair helps to regulate his body temperature.

**or your baby**

Make a list of your hopes and dreams for your baby and have your partner do the same. Compare lists and see where your goals for your child intersect.

**our body today**

Don't be surprised if your thoughts turn to sex today. As your morning sickness wanes and your breasts and vagina continue to benefit from increased sensitivity and blood flow, your libido may pick up.

**or your body**

This can be a great time to reconnect with your partner (who you may have kept at a distance until now due to sickness, discomfort, or just plain grouchiness). A renewed physical closeness with your loved one may be just the thing your mind, body, and relationship need. While you're at it, take advantage of the freedom you still have to enjoy a variety of sex positions. Once your belly becomes large, your options will become more limited.

How I Feel

My Thoughts

Week 11 Weigh-in:_____lbs

# Day 193    Date _____

**Your baby today**

Your baby's head has become more proportional to his body. It went from being half th[e] length of his body to about a third the length of his body.

*For your baby*

You may want to look into a savings account called a 529 plan today. While your baby['s] college education is far off into the future, it may take you years to save enough for tuitio[n]. The 529 helps you save for the rising cost of higher education without being taxed on th[e] money you earn.

**Your body today**

You are busting at the seams of your non-maternity pants and your regular shirts are startin[g] to feel like half shirts. Even your bras are no longer doing their job.

*For your body*

Time to get out there and splurge a little on some maternity basics like plain colore[d] shirts and jeans or basic black pants. Get more for your money by shopping at any of th[e] large department stores that now carry maternity clothes. While it may be tempting to bu[y] clothes that fit you perfectly now, it's smarter to buy one or two sizes larger to get use o[ut] of each item.

*How I Feel* _____

_____

_____

*My Thoughts* _____

_____

_____

# Day 192    Date _____

**Your baby today**

If your baby is a girl, she already has 2 million eggs in her ovaries.

*For your baby*

Add a heaping portion of steamed broccoli to your next meal and build up your calciu[m] stores for baby. Not a big fan of broccoli? Melting a slice of cheese on top will add some extr[a] calcium and appeal.

**Your body today**

You may be gaining a little weight all over or it may be concentrated in a ball shape o[r] in front. Either way, some people will think that your weight gain is a clue to the gend[er] of your baby.

*For your body*

Have fun guessing the gender of your baby based on how you "wear" your pregnanc[y]. Traditional thinking assumes that women with a low, basketball-shaped bump will have [a] boy, while women who carry their bump higher and gain weight in other places will have [a] girl. There's no scientific credence to these theories, but in the absence of an ultrasound an[d] an expert opinion, they are all anyone has to go on.

How I Feel _____

My Thoughts _____

**Your baby today**

Fingerprints—completely unique in their design—now decorate the tiny tips of your baby's fingers.

**For your baby**

Flaxseed and flaxseed oil have an estrogenic effect on the body that may or may not harm an unborn child. In several studies, rats exposed to flaxseed in utero have exhibited sexual abnormalities. If flaxseed is currently part of your diet, you may want to remove it completely until more is known about its effects on human hormones.

**Your body today**

Time to consider whether you want to know your baby's gender. In just a few weeks, you will have an ultrasound test to check the general health of your baby and (if you choose) to find out the baby's gender.

**For your body**

Still unsure? Here are two arguments for finding out the gender of your baby and two reasons against: Knowing your baby's gender may help to deepen your bond with him/her during pregnancy. Finding out also means you don't have to suspend your curiosity for another 190 days. On the other hand, waiting until delivery day may provide the extra incentive you need to get through hard labor. Waiting to know your baby's gender also allows you to experience that classic, "It's a girl!" or "It's a boy!" moment after all your hard work. Don't rush this very personal decision. Take time to discuss it with your partner.

How I Feel _____

My Thoughts _____

**Your baby today**

Your baby is getting cuter every day. Not only is her body catching up to her head, but her eyes have moved closer together on her face and her ears are in their proper positions.

*For your baby*

Hooray! You have reached the end of your 1st trimester and carried your baby through the riskiest period of her early life. The chance of miscarriage (about 15 to 20 percent in healthy women) has now drastically decreased to between 1 and 5 percent, so breathe a sigh of relief and keep doing what you've been doing.

**Your body today**

You may start to feel like your old self again today. Maybe you didn't have to roll down all the windows on your drive to work this morning, maybe you were able to enjoy a food that normally churns your stomach, or maybe your mood and energy level are improving.

*For your body*

Nausea does not go away magically one day, but slowly subsides. You may not even notice it until it's gone, but you are already on the path to feeling better. If you escaped morning sickness altogether, then you no longer have to feel self-conscious telling people that you feel just fine.

*How I Feel* _____

_____

*My Thoughts* _____

_____

_____

I never really had morning sickness: I had afternoon and evening sickness. I was plagued with constant headaches and nausea that didn't go away until my sixteenth week. Too long in my opinion, but after that I was a whole new person: My energy was back and I could enjoy all kinds of good foods again.

—Kerry G., mother of 6-week-old Shannon

# Daddy's Turn

Daddy's Thoughts and Feelings

Happiest Moments So Far
_____
_____
_____
_____
_____

My Concerns or Fears
_____
_____
_____
_____
_____

My Hopes and Dreams for the Baby
_____
_____
_____
_____

A Message for My Pregnant Wife/Partner
_____
_____
_____
_____
_____

My Guess as to the Baby's Gender
_____

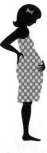

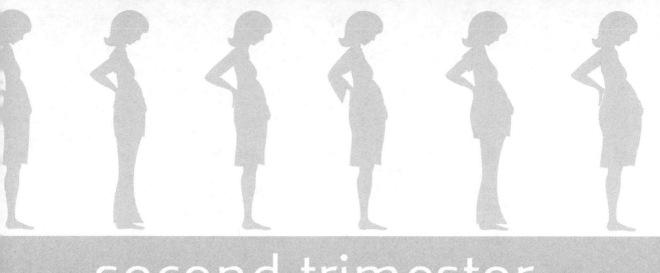

# second trimester

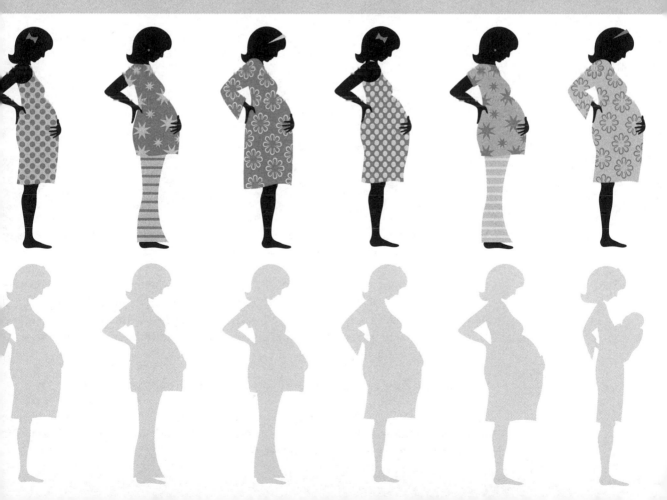

# Day 189    Date _____

**Your baby today**

Your baby's heart is beating at about twice the rate of yours today.

**For your baby**

Because a baby is deprived of some oxygen during contractions, his or her heart rate monitored all through labor. If it drops too low or if the baby shows signs of stress durin labor, changing positions (lying on your left side or resting on your hands and knee may help it return to normal. To foresee any heart rate issues, your medical provider ma recommend a contraction stress test much later in your pregnancy to test the baby's hea rate during simulated contractions.

**Your body today**

You may experience some bleeding or spotting after sex.

**For your body**

Most spotting and light bleeding after sex is nothing to worry about. Deep penetration ca irritate and break the sensitive blood vessels at the tip of your cervix and cause spotting bleeding. If the bleeding continues or gets heavier, call your medical provider. Otherwis opt for a kinder, gentler sex position next time.

*How I Feel* _____

_____

_____

*My Thoughts* _____

_____

_____

# Day 188    Date _____

**Your baby today**

Your baby is experimenting with more fine-tuned movement like bending her wrists ar toes, flexing her hands, and bending her knees.

**For your baby**

Step foot into a baby gear store and you'll probably be overwhelmed by all of the equipme available. If you're not sure where to begin, ask an experienced mom to give you a list of th items she absolutely could not have lived without in those first few months. Gather a few these lists from friends and you'll be much more prepared to stock up on the essentials ar register for baby shower gifts.

**Your body today**

Your palms and the pads of your feet may have a reddish tint and itch a little.

**For your body**

This skin condition, called "palmar erythema" is specific to pregnancy and will disappe after delivery. To relieve itching, soak a facecloth in a mixture of cornstarch, baking sod and water and apply it to hands and feet.

How I Feel _____

My Thoughts _____

## Day 187    Date _____

**Your baby today**

Your child's nervous system has started functioning, meaning his brain can now relay important messages to various parts of his body.

**For your baby**

While pastels are often the nursery décor of choice, consider decorating your baby's room in bright, contrasting colors as those are the shades he will be able to see and appreciate first.

**Your body today**

Your dreams may be getting more bizarre and may start to center on pregnancy and babies. Many women have nightmares about being bad mothers, having unhealthy babies, or being abandoned by their mates and having to take care of the baby on their own.

**For your body**

Some of your worst fears about having a baby will inevitably manifest themselves in your dreams. Don't read into your nightmares too much. Allow them to serve their purpose: to highlight your hidden anxieties and force you to confront them.

How I Feel _____

My Thoughts _____

## Day 186    Date _____

**Your baby today**

Your baby has a light sprinkling of hair on his head today.

**For your baby**

Want to get an idea of how much hair your baby will be born with? According to an old wives' tale, the more heartburn you endure during pregnancy, the thicker your baby's hair will be at birth.

Week 12 Weigh-in: ____lbs

| Your body today | Just as your baby is sprouting new hair, so are you—sometimes in places where it's not at all welcome. |
|---|---|
| *For your body* | If you're getting unwanted hairs on your face, stomach, back or legs, you have something in common with many other pregnant women. Sadly, your tweezers may be working overtime for the next 185 days. On a happier note, leg hair often grows slower during pregnancy, allowing you to go longer without shaving your legs. |

How I Feel

My Thoughts

# Day 185  Date _____

| Your baby today | Your baby may be holding or playing with his umbilical cord today, which is now about the same length as his body (3-4 inches). |
|---|---|
| *For your baby* | You may have told your boss by now that you are expecting a baby. If you haven't yet discussed the terms of your maternity leave, make sure you're properly prepared for this important discussion. First, do your research and get a copy of your company's maternity leave policy. Then, write down your ideal scenario: the date you want to stop working, the amount of paid and unpaid leave you expect, the date you want to return to work, and any other details that are important to you. While your company may have a standard policy for maternity leave, there is usually some room for negotiation. |
| Your body today | Your uterus has grown from about the size of a pear to the size of a grapefruit. The top of it, also called your "fundus," is now bulging just above your pubic bone. |
| *For your body* | For a healthy snack that feels like dessert, try dipping some whole grain crackers in vanilla or strawberry low-fat yogurt. |

How I Feel

My Thoughts

**our baby today**

Your baby is getting a longer neck and cute little cheeks! He's about the size of a kiwi today.

**or your baby**

Coming down with a cold or a cough during pregnancy will not harm your baby, but alcohol and other ingredients in common cold medicines could do harm. Talk to your doctor before taking any over-the-counter cold medicine.

**our body today**

Even if you avoided eating fatty, greasy foods today, you may still experience some heartburn.

**or your body**

Heartburn can occur all through pregnancy, thanks to the effect of hormones on your digestive system and the pressure that your growing uterus puts on your stomach. While fatty and fried foods are typical culprits, you may not realize that foods containing citrus, tomato, chocolate, peppermint, or pepper can also bring on a bad case of heartburn. Avoid these items and you may spare yourself some discomfort after meals.

How I Feel _____

My Thoughts _____

**our baby today**

Today your baby is using his new facial muscles to frown, squint, and pucker his lips. He has a variety of facial expressions now, some of which may resemble yours or your partner's.

**or your baby**

If you're going to be gardening, throw on some gloves to avoid exposing the baby to any toxins in the soil. Lead, insecticides, animal feces, and fertilizer could all pose a health risk to your child.

**our body today**

If you experience pain or burning when you urinate today, it may be a sign of a urinary tract infection.

**or your body**

Urinary tract infections are more common in pregnancy, and like any infection they pose health risks to you and your baby. If you do experience the symptoms above, or if you notice any blood in your urine, bring them to your medical provider's attention immediately.

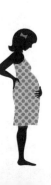

How I Feel _____

My Thoughts _____
_____

## Day 182   Date _____

**Your baby today**

Your placenta has started to produce heat that raises your body temperature and keeps yo[u] baby's body temperature steady at about 1 degree warmer than yours.

*For your baby*

Because your body temperature is so closely tied to your baby's, continue to keep yours at [a] safe level (100 degrees or less). This might mean a shorter morning run when it's especia[lly] hot outside or a dose of acetaminophen to bring down a high fever.

**Your body today**

The placenta is now your main progesterone supplier. The surge of hormones it provides [is] boosting your metabolism and may have you feeling happier and more energetic.

*For your body*

While some women endure morning sickness throughout their entire pregnancy, most a[re] liberated from their nausea by this week or next. Take advantage of your increased ener[gy] and better mood to tackle projects or errands that have been languishing on your to-do li[st] for months.

How I Feel _____
_____

My Thoughts _____
_____
_____

## Day 181   Date _____

**Your baby today**

Today your baby has the beginnings of eyebrows!

*For your baby*

Want to do your baby and the environment a favor? Splurge on eco-friendly diapers. Wh[ile] diaper recycling hasn't really caught on, there are a few popular brands of diapers o[ut] there made from unbleached cotton. Using unbleached diapers helps keep harmful an[d] unnecessary chemicals (like chlorine) off your baby's body and out of our soil and rivers.

**our body today**

If you were overweight before your pregnancy, you may have already been warned by your doctor that you're at greater risk for blood clots, hypertension, and gestational diabetes during pregnancy.

**or your body**

Regular exercise and careful attention to the extra calories you're consuming help minimize your health risks if you're overweight. Aim to gain between 15 and 25 pounds instead of the usual 25 to 35.

*How I Feel* _____

_____

*My Thoughts* _____

_____

_____

# Day 180    Date _____

**our baby today**

An increase in the amount of amniotic fluid in his gestational sac has allowed your baby to swim about with more ease and comfort. He now has about a quart of fluid to support and suspend his fast-growing body.

**or your baby**

If other moms offer you their used baby gear and clothes, take advantage! Saving your money on a few pieces of baby gear may allow you to splurge on that one big-ticket item you've been eyeing. Likewise, an extra bag of hand-me-down clothes will prove useful if your baby spits up a lot. Who wants to do laundry every day?

**our body today**

You may feel your baby moving today for the first time! It's easy to dismiss these first movements as gas bubbles or indigestion, but soon you'll be able to tell the two apart with ease.

**or your body**

Don't be alarmed if you don't feel the baby moving yet. For some women, it takes another 30 days to be sure that those lower belly flutters are actually the baby. Feeling your baby "quickening" can be very emotional and may make up for the sacrifices you are making now as a mom.

*How I Feel* _____

_____

*My Thoughts* _____

_____

Week 13 Weigh-in:_____lbs

## Day 179    Date _____

**Your baby today**

Your baby's bone density is steadily increasing and his hands can now clench into tiny fist

*For your baby*

Enjoy a dinner of fresh salmon and asparagus tonight. Salmon is a great source of omega vitamins and selenium for your baby's developing brain while the chromium in asparag is thought to stave off gestational diabetes. Light a candle and make a toast (with yo sparkling grape juice) to the health of your baby.

**Your body today**

If you started at a normal weight, you have probably put on about 5 pounds pregnancy weight.

*For your body*

Stepping onto a scale at each prenatal appointment can put your weight under uncomfortab scrutiny. If you're self-conscious about your changing weight, keep in mind that this is one those rare times in life when weight gain is an admirable accomplishment. Tell your partn or husband about your insecurities and ask them to remind you from time to time th weight gain means you are simply doing your job.

How I Feel _____

_____

My Thoughts _____

_____

## Day 178    Date _____

**Your baby today**

Your baby does not yet sleep. His activity level stays fairly consistent throughout the day ar night and he seldom rests in one position for more than seven minutes.

When the time comes to paint the nursery, leave the job to someone else. Breathing in paint fumes could be harmful to your baby, though a lot is still unknown about the exact effects. Keep your home well ventilated when painting is underway and avoid using spray paints, as they disperse even more potentially dangerous particles into the air.

**our body today**

If you are used to sleeping on your stomach, your belly may now prevent you from doing so. Sleeping on your side, though recommended, may not be easy at first.

**or your body**

It's time to invest in a pregnancy support pillow or to employ the use of extra pillows to support your new side-sleeping habit. You may need to sample a few different pillow combinations before settling on the best one for you.

How I Feel ........................................................................................................................

........................................................................................................................

My Thoughts ....................................................................................................................

........................................................................................................................

# Day 177 Date _____

**our baby today**

Your baby's umbilical cord now circulates up to 20 quarts of fluid a day. The baby's steady flow of blood straightens the cord and prevents it from becoming permanently knotted or tangled.

**or your baby**

Studies in animals have found a link between diets high in nitrates (a preservative used in hot dogs, bacon, etc.) and low-birth-weight babies. If you love hot dogs, but are worried about the questionable effect of nitrates on your baby's growth, look for nitrate-free hot dogs at your supermarket or natural food store. Nitrate-free hot dogs may still contain some nitrates in the form of celery water, but nitrates from vegetables are not believed to be harmful to your baby.

**our body today**

You may find yourself sweating more than usual as you hike up a flight of stairs today. The increased blood volume in your body helps support your growing baby, but it may also cause you to perspire more.

**or your body**

Roll on an extra layer of deodorant, dress in light layers so you can remove a layer if needed, and drink lots of water to replenish the water lost by sweating.

How I Feel ........................................................................................................................

........................................................................................................................

My Thoughts ....................................................................................................................

## Day 176    Date _____

### Your baby today
Your baby weighs about 2 ounces today and is almost 5 inches long from his hea to his rump!

### For your baby
Don't be afraid to start talking to, or singing to, your baby at this stage of pregnancy. H ears are still developing, but he can hear a variety of sounds already and may find you voice soothing. If you get sick of hearing your own voice, consider playing some music f him instead.

### Your body today
If you're like some women, you may experience "warm-up" contractions, also known a Braxton Hicks, as early as today. The muscles in your uterus will cramp and tighten and th surface of your stomach will feel as hard as a rock.

### For your body
If you experience this form of cramping later in the day or in the evening, it may be th you're working your body too hard and need to rest. Treat yourself to as much relaxation a possible and see if the contractions subside. If the contractions are getting more painful ar coming more often, call your doctor of midwife immediately.

How I Feel _____

_____

_____

My Thoughts _____

_____

_____

## Day 175    Date _____

### Your baby today
More and more of your baby's cells are being shed into his fluid surrounding These cells, if extracted, offer incredible insight into his genetics and can reve chromosomal abnormalities.

### For your baby
If your pregnancy is considered high-risk, your doctor may suggest a procedure called a amniocentesis around this time. If you do have this procedure done, a small sample amniotic fluid will be extracted from your baby's gestational sac. The results will determine with a high level of accuracy—whether your child has a number of common disorde including Down syndrome, Trisomy 21, cystic fibrosis, or spina bifida.

### Your body today
Because there are so many more screening and diagnostic tests available to today pregnant women, you may be confused or overwhelmed trying to decide which tests a right for you.

Speaking with your doctor about the risks (if any) associated with each test and the value of the test results (in terms of what can be done for a baby if the tests come back positive) may help steer you in a clearer direction. You should also consider your partner's perspective and check with your health insurance company to see which tests are covered under your plan.

*How I Feel* _____

_____

*My Thoughts* _____

_____

> At my 20-week ultrasound, I was told that my baby's bowel was echogenic, meaning it was showing up brighter than normal on the ultrasound. This can be nothing or it can be a soft marker for Down syndrome, cystic fibrosis, or some other chromosomal abnormality. We decided to go ahead and do an amniocentesis to find out for sure. Luckily, everything came back normal and the baby is fine, but there were some stressful weeks of worrying in between.
>
> —Olga, mother of 8-month-old Sven

## Day 174 Date _____

**Your baby today**

Your baby now has an active immune system, though he still needs your antibodies to help protect him from bacteria and viruses.

**For your baby**

If you've been putting off calling the exterminator about a mouse or rat problem, time to stop procrastinating. According to the Centers for Disease Control, interacting with any kind of rodent during pregnancy (including pet hamsters and guinea pigs) could put your baby at risk of getting a serious virus called lymphocytic choriomeningitis, or LCMV. For more pregnancy advice from the CDC, go to http://www.cdc.gov/ncbddd/bd/abc.htm.

Week 14 Weigh-in:____lbs

| Your body today | You may feel a sharp pain in your lower abdomen if you twist, turn, laugh, or even get up too quickly today. This is known as round ligament pain. |
|---|---|
| *For your body* | Your growing uterus is causing your stomach muscles to stretch in a new way. If you do experience round ligament pain, the best thing to do is relax in one position until the pain subsides. If it continues, try soaking in a warm bath. Persistent abdominal pain should be reported to your doctor or midwife. |

How I Feel _____

_____

My Thoughts _____

_____

## Day 173  Date _____

| Your baby today | If you could see all the rolling and stretching and kicking your baby is doing today, you'd see that she is becoming much more coordinated. |
|---|---|
| *For your baby* | Make a healthy trail mix today complete with almonds, sunflower seeds, pumpkin seeds and your favorite dried fruit. You'll get a helping of healthy fats to lower your cholesterol and the baby will get a dose of the nutrients she needs. |
| Your body today | Because your weight is distributed differently now and your bulging belly is putting you slightly off balance, you may have an aching back today. |
| *For your body* | Avoid standing or sitting for too long in one position. If you sit in front of a computer for long periods of time, set a reminder to take short walks around the office and get you body moving. Prenatal yoga classes and other exercises that improve your muscle tone and posture are a great way to avoid some of the aches and pains of pregnancy. |

How I Feel _____

_____

My Thoughts _____

_____

## Day 172  Date _____

| Your baby today | Your baby's arms and legs are now longer and thinner and her little pot belly is getting more and more pronounced. |
|---|---|

Traveling by plane is perfectly safe for you and your baby at this point. Because commercial planes are pressurized, you won't be depriving the baby of any oxygen. While most airlines will let you fly up until 36 weeks, vacationing or traveling for business before the end of your second trimester is preferable. If you do fly, be sure to get up and walk around every hour to increase circulation and prevent blood clots from forming.

### Your body today

You may be craving some quality time with your significant other before the baby arrives. Now may be the perfect occasion for a "babymoon," one last excursion before the demands of parenthood take precedence. Schedule a night or a weekend away and savor this unique time in your relationship.

### For your body

If you miss that occasional glass of beer or wine, make it your mission to find a mocktail, or non-alcoholic cocktail, you enjoy almost as much. Mix your favorite juice with seltzer water or experiment at home with mocktail recipes you find online. Try a glass of orange juice with a splash of grenadine; drop some lime juice in your cola, or grab some margarita mix at the store and enjoy it without the alcohol.

How I Feel _____

My Thoughts _____

---

## Day 171          Date

### Your baby today

Your baby is swallowing and excreting amniotic fluid and hiccupping silently in your womb.

### For your baby

A baby needs lots of protein and iron to develop. Whip up a spinach omelet today and combine the protein power of eggs with the iron present in spinach. Other iron-rich foods include red meat, poultry, fish, pasta and cereal. Try enjoying them with citrus fruits, green peppers, or other foods high in vitamin C to maximize the amount of iron your body absorbs.

### Your body today

You may feel gassy, tired, or sick to your stomach after a meal today as your sluggish digestive system tries to keep up with your food intake.

### For your body

While it may seem strange at first, don't drink anything with your next meal. Drink between meals and you may notice that your heartburn and indigestion symptoms ease up.

How I Feel _____

My Thoughts _____

## Day 170  Date _____

**Your baby today**

Increased calcium absorption is making your baby's bones harder and stronger. His joint are all in working order today.

*For your baby*

You may want to research and read customer reviews of popular baby swings, highchairs slings, bouncy seats, cribs, strollers, and car seats. Doing your homework ahead of time wi keep you from feeling overwhelmed when it comes time to go shopping or register at particular store.

**Your body today**

Hopefully, you are starting to understand what they mean by that pregnancy "glow Increased blood circulation in the second trimester may bring an extra flush of color to you face while increased oil production may give your skin a healthy sheen.

*For your body*

Enjoy the compliments you get at this stage of pregnancy as well as the added attention. someone offers you his seat, take it. Being pregnant is not always an easy job, so reap th rewards when you can.

How I Feel _____

_____

_____

_____

My Thoughts _____

_____

_____

_____

## Day 169  Date _____

**Your baby today**

Your baby would have a hard time keeping his or her gender a secret from a traine ultrasound technician today.

*For your baby*

You don't have to wait until you know the gender to start buying clothes or nurse décor for your little one. You don't even have to limit yourself to an endless array of pa greens and yellows. Reds, oranges, and shades of tan are just a few of today's popula gender-neutral options.

**Your body today**

Soon you'll be able to see what's been taking place inside your body over the last 169 days. you have an ultrasound scheduled for this month, you may be eager to find out if your bab is healthy and whether you're having a girl or a boy.

Brace yourself for the possibility that you may leave your ultrasound appointment with only a guess as to the baby's gender. Some ultrasound technicians don't like to make a definite call unless the genitalia are unmistakable. You may also have a mischievous (or shy) baby who keeps his/her legs crossed during the entire procedure.

How I Feel

My Thoughts

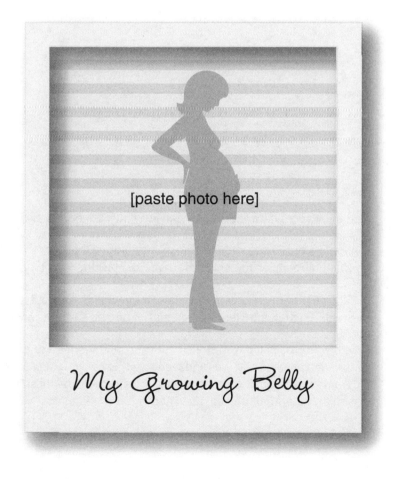

[paste photo here]

*My Growing Belly*

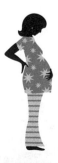

**Your baby today**

Your baby is starting to get his baby fat today! His face and body will soon fill out and th extra accumulation of fat tissue beneath will help regulate his body temperature when h enters the outside world.

*For your baby*

A snack of fiber-rich crackers and cheese will give you the protein your baby needs to buil every one of his cells and the fiber you need for a healthy digestive system.

**Your body today**

Your growing uterus is pushing your intestines upward and moving them to the sid of your body.

*For your body*

If you experience constipation as a result of your overcrowded intestines, try trading you morning orange juice for a juice with more fiber (like prune or pear juice). Be sure to drin lots of water and move your bowels when the urge first strikes.

How I Feel _____

_____

_____

_____

My Thoughts _____

_____

_____

**Your baby today**

Your baby's eyes have lashes now and are much larger, but they are still closed.

*For your baby*

Ask your parents for something from your childhood that you can add to the baby's nursery. favorite doll, blanket, toy, or keepsake may be just the right touch to personalize the room

**Your body today**

Weight gain and changes in your blood circulation can put extra pressure on your le muscles. You may experience leg cramps or muscle seizures in your legs today as a result

*For your body*

Do a few exercises today to stretch out your calf muscles. For example: While standing, li your weight onto your tip-toes and then slowly lower your heel back down again. If a painfu leg cramp strikes, apply a heating pad to the area until the muscles relax. Sleeping with you legs slightly elevated can help prevent nighttime cramping.

How I Feel _____

_____

_____

_____

# Day 166 Date _____

**Your baby today**

The individual bones in your baby's hands and feet are well developed now. Ten little fingernails and ten little toenails have grown on the ends of his fingers and toes.

**For your baby**

Notify your doctor of any herbal supplements you are currently taking. Little is known about their effects during pregnancy, since their safety and use is not regulated by the U.S. Food and Drug Administration. In light of their association with birth defects in laboratory animals, supplements like gingko biloba and ginseng are best avoided during pregnancy.

**Your body today**

Minor aches and pains can start to become an annoyance around this time. Today, you may feel the need to escape from all the changes that are happening to your body.

**For your body**

Swimming is a great way to feel lighter (if only temporarily), keep from gaining extra weight, and alleviate the physical nuisances of pregnancy. If your gym doesn't have a pool, consider joining a new one or tag along with a friend with access to a pool. You'll be amazed at how relieved you'll feel gliding weightlessly through water.

How I Feel _____

My Thoughts _____

# Day 165 Date _____

**Your baby today**

Your baby enters a new stage of maturity today because he has developed something called proprioception, an awareness of his own body parts. Thanks to advancements in his cerebellum, when he touches his mouth or knee or face today, he may realize that it's connected to his body.

**For your baby**

Now that your baby is starting to form his identity, it may be a good time to start narrowing down that list of baby names. Reserve an hour of time tonight with your partner to discuss any favorites that you have in common. Don't get upset if you can't agree on many names in the beginning. Compromise will probably play a key role in this process.

**Your body today**

It's not uncommon to experience rectal discomfort at this stage of pregnancy or to see bloo[d] when you wipe after a bowel movement. Hemorrhoids, varicose veins in the rectum tha[t] swell and bleed, can flare up due to pressure from your enlarged uterus and an increase i[n] your blood volume.

**For your body**

Hemorrhoids are yet another reason to avoid sleeping on your back at night, as this will onl[y] increase the amount of pressure on the enlarged veins. If a cold compress and a warm bat[h] of baking soda and water don't help with the pain and itching, check with your doctor abou[t] trying topical hemorrhoid ointments.

*How I Feel* _____

*My Thoughts* _____

_____

# Day 164  Date _____

**Your baby today**

Your baby's circulatory system and urinary system are fully functioning today. His umbilica[l] cord is getting thicker and stronger all the time.

**For your baby**

If you've already gone shopping for your baby, you may be wondering about the organi[c] cotton bedding and clothing trend. Most cotton carries some trace of the pesticides used t[o] grow it. Those who are concerned about the effects of these toxins on their baby's sensitiv[e] skin—and those who prefer the look and feel—will pay extra for organic cotton items.

**Your body today**

You are probably amazed by how hungry you feel all the time now that you are 164 day[s] into your pregnancy. You may also be amazed that your cravings have steered you in ne[w] directions. Spicy food was never a palate pleaser before, but now you can't get enough!

**For your body**

Get your extra 300 calories today with an assortment of fresh vegetables dipped in hummu[s] or low-calorie dressing.

*How I Feel* _____

*My Thoughts* _____

_____

# Day 163  Date _____

**Your baby today**

Today your baby's heart will pump about 50 pints of blood through his body.

**or your baby**

Now is a good time to invest in some books about newborn health, infant sleep "training," or breastfeeding. You won't have much time when the baby comes to brush up on these key topics, so educate yourself now to prepare for the challenges ahead.

**our body today**

An intense chocolate or ice cream craving may strike today. As much as you try to ignore it, it keeps coming back.

**or your body**

Treat yourself to a decadent dessert today and enjoy every bite of it. Just be sure to eat it at least a few hours before bed so that indigestion and heartburn don't disturb your sleep.

*How I Feel*

*My Thoughts*

> I swam a lot during my first pregnancy because the water was the only place I didn't feel like a whale. Ironic, right?
>
> —Chantal, mother of 8-week-old Willem

# Day 162  Date _____

**our baby today**

Your baby is over 5½ inches long and weighs about 4 ounces today.

**or your baby**

If you've never been a fan of fruits and vegetables, now is the time to develop a taste for them. Get a juicer and try making homemade fruit-and-veggie juice blends, like carrot-pomegranate or apple-celery. You'll benefit from nutrients and much-needed fiber, along with a healthy snack.

**our body today**

You may feel some pain in your back or lower abdomen when you lift something that's too heavy today.

**or your body**

Because you're now prone to round ligament and back pain, avoid lifting anything over 30 pounds. If you do any lifting, use your leg muscles as much as possible and hold the item close to your body as you lift.

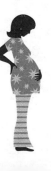

How I Feel _____

My Thoughts _____

# Day 161 Date _____

**Your baby today**

It may not be adorable to imagine, but your baby's skull remains open today to allow for hi developing brain.

*For your baby*

You may find that you get a lot of unsolicited advice from friends, family, and strangers abou what you should and shouldn't do for the sake of your unborn baby. Your doctor or midwif should be the source you trust most to make all of these decisions. After that, trust you instincts and try not to get overwhelmed by all the dos and don'ts of pregnancy.

**Your body today**

Hunger may come on quickly today and hit you like a Mack truck. When it does, be ready.

*For your body*

When hunger strikes, you'll be tempted to grab the food that's quickest and easiest. If fa food is a constant temptation during your pregnancy, try keeping some granola bars or cerea bars in your desk drawer or in your cabinets. They're quick and easy to indulge in, and the may hold off your hunger pangs long enough for you to prepare or order a healthy meal.

How I Feel _____

My Thoughts _____

I must have done at least three Google searches to find out if eating blue cheese dressing was okay during pregnancy. In the end I didn't eat it because I read too many "don't do its" online and who wants that guilt?

—Carolyn T., mother of 7-month-old Alex

# Day 160    Date _____

**Your baby today**

Some of your baby's nerves are getting a protective layer called myelin today. Myelin helps the messages from your baby's brain travel efficiently from one nerve cell to the next.

**For your baby**

Now that you're driving for two, be sure to buckle up every time you get in the car. Wear the lap belt under your belly, tight against your hips, to protect yourself and minimize the danger to your baby if you should become involved in an accident.

**Your body today**

Now that you are able to (or nearing the day when you will) find out the gender of your baby, you may realize that you or your partner are rooting for one gender over another.

**For your body**

Preferring a boy or a girl baby is nothing to feel guilty about. Most people have an easier time picturing themselves with one or the other. If you find out the gender early, you will have plenty of time to get used to the idea of something different. By the time delivery day rolls around, the only thing most parents are rooting for is a healthy baby.

How I Feel _____

_____

My Thoughts _____

_____

# Day 159    Date _____

**Your baby today**

Tiny air sacs are beginning to develop inside your baby's lungs today. They're called alveoli, and they'll come in handy when he breathes air for the first time.

**For your baby**

It's still unknown why childhood allergies and asthma are on the rise, but some studies cite high levels of stress during pregnancy as a contributing factor. Try to relax as much as possible with soothing music, warm baths, and massage. Other contributing factors may be the time of year your baby is born and whether allergies and asthma run in your family.

**Your body today**

Your blood pressure may be lower than normal today and could trigger feelings of dizziness or lightheadedness.

**For your body**

Stop whatever you're doing and rest until the dizzy spell or lightheadedness passes. Halfway into pregnancy, many women experience symptoms of a drop in blood pressure. Your doctor or midwife should be monitoring your blood pressure at every visit—he or she will let you know if your reading is too low or too high.

Week 16 Weigh-in:_____lbs

## Day 158    Date _____

**Your baby today**
Your baby's eyes have finally migrated to their final position at the front of her head. It wi be another 6 weeks or so before they are developed enough to open.

**Your baby today**
If you have a family pet, you may have concerns about how you will manage a peacefu relationship between the newborn baby and your pet. If you have a dog that shows an signs of aggression, especially toward children, consider hiring a dog trainer immediately t address the problem before the baby arrives.

**Your body today**
The fullness in your breasts and lower belly are now becoming obvious. You may also fin that you are gaining weight in other places (face, bottom, thighs) and that your diaphragr is slowly expanding.

*For your body*
You may feel like it's obvious that you're pregnant, but don't be surprised or insulted if takes a few more months before people feel comfortable bringing it up. Soon enough, ever cashier, hairdresser, and salesperson you meet will take one look at your figure and want t discuss your pregnancy.

How I Feel _____

My Thoughts _____

_____

_____

## Day 157    Date _____

**Your baby today**
If you have a little girl, her fallopian tubes and uterus are now in their right place. If you hav a boy, his prostate is beginning to form and will one day distribute semen and sperm.

*For your baby*
If there is a chance that you're having a boy, you may want to talk to your partner an your doctor about the risks and benefits of circumcision. You may be surprised to find ou that while 50 to 60 percent of boys in the U.S. are circumcised, there are few, if any, healt reasons for the procedure. The American Academy of Pediatrics states that while dat indicates some medical benefits from circumcision, the data is not sufficient to recommen the procedure.

| Your body today | Despite eating healthy, you may find that you're gaining weight more rapidly than you'd like. |
|---|---|
| For your body | Fruit juices are often a hidden source of extra calories. If you're drinking more than a few cups of fruit juice every day, consider switching to vegetable juice. It packs just as many nutrients but has fewer calories. Another option is to substitute your regular fruit juice for a lower-calorie alternative, like grapefruit juice. |

How I Feel _____

_____

_____

My Thoughts _____

_____

# Day 156  Date _____

| Your baby today | Punching and kicking are two ways that your baby will exercise her growing body today. |
|---|---|
| For your baby | Educate yourself on SIDS (sudden infant death syndrome) in the months to come. About 3 in 1,000 infants between the age of 1 and 3 months die inexplicably during sleep. Although the cause of SIDS is still unknown, it is tied to long pauses in the baby's breathing. You can reduce the risk of SIDS by always placing your baby to sleep on her back. Clear the baby's sleep area of any stuffed animals, blankets, or suffocation hazards and do not cover the baby with a blanket while she sleeps. For more information on SIDS, go to http://www.sids.org/nprevent.htm. |
| Your body today | Your hormones have gone haywire and you find yourself getting easily frustrated today. |
| For your body | Treat yourself to a little exercise to ease your body of excess stress and tension. If you know of any other expecting mothers, it may help your motivation to partner up a few times a week for a long walk or a yoga class. |

How I Feel _____

_____

My Thoughts _____

_____

_____

_____

# Day 155   Date _____

**Your baby today**

Today your baby could be as long as 6 inches from head to rump and may weigh abou[t] 5¼ ounces.

**For your baby**

Disposable diapers are still the top choice for today's busy or working parent, but the cos[t] can be considerable. Cloth diapers are a more frugal, environmentally friendly, (and, some say, leak-resistant) alternative to disposables. Moms who use them are willing to take on a[?] few extra loads of laundry every week to reap the benefits. If you like the environmental[ly] friendly aspect of cloth diapers but don't welcome the extra work, look for a diaper servic[e] in your area.

**Your body today**

You may feel a little down or depressed today and wonder if it's pregnancy-related.

**For your body**

The alternating joys and rigors of pregnancy are fertile ground for depression and anxiet[y] disorders. While mood swings are perfectly normal, about 1 in 10 moms-to-be suffer fro[m] serious depression. If you find that you are lethargic, apathetic, have no appetite, or fee[l] depressed or anxious most of the day, see a specialist and make sure you get the treatmen[t] you need.

How I Feel _____

_____

My Thoughts _____

_____

# Day 154   Date _____

**Your baby today**

Your baby may react to a car alarm, a slamming door, or blaring music by becoming mor[e] active. He or she is beginning to hear more and more of the outside world.

**For your baby**

Play your favorite music for your baby while riding in the car or relaxing at home. Sing alon[g] and allow your baby to be soothed by your voice.

**Your body today**

In your first trimester, you were visiting the bathroom every hour. Now that your thirst i[s] unquenchable, the water cooler has become your best friend.

**For your body**

Drinking at least eight glasses of water a day is always recommended, and is even mor[e] essential when you're pregnant. The water you drink is used to build new tissue, facilitat[e] digestion, and carry nutrients throughout your body. To be sure you meet this dail[y] requirement, keep a water bottle in your car, on your desk, and by your bedside at home.

## Day 153    Date _____

**Your baby today**

Your baby could be sitting in a yoga position with her back straight and her legs crossed. She can flip and arch her back and extend her arms and legs with ease.

**For your baby**

Try to engage your baby in a game today: Wait for a kick or movement from within and tap the spot on your abdomen where you felt it happen. See if the baby responds with a second movement and respond to that movement with another gentle pat. Enjoy the feeling of communicating with your child.

**Your body today**

Suddenly, you can feel your baby moving! You're bonding with the baby more than ever, but your partner is a little jealous.

**For your body**

Involving your partner in this recent milestone will help him foster his own unique connection with the baby. Don't be disappointed if he doesn't always feel every kick and flutter you can feel. He may just be content to rest his hand on your belly for a while and "get to know" his son or daughter.

## Day 152    Date _____

**Your baby today**

Your baby's sense of touch is now one of his most refined senses. He will caress his own face or body today and may rub the soles of his feet together.

**For your baby**

If you are still choosing your baby registry items, don't forget to add skin care items like gentle moisturizing lotion, baby shampoo, and baby oil (for giving your newborn relaxing massages).

Week 17 Weigh-in: _____ lbs

| Your body today | You may feel guilty about indulging in more sweets than healthy nutrients today. |
|---|---|

| For your body | While it's important to eat a healthy diet to support your pregnancy, expect to have some days where you satisfy your taste buds instead of your daily nutritional requirements. Lose the guilt and make a plan to eat healthier tomorrow. |
|---|---|

*How I Feel* _____

_____

*My Thoughts* _____

_____

## Day 151    Date _____

| Your baby today | If you are having identical or fraternal twins, they are starting to physically interact with each other in a playful, and sometimes even competitive, way. One will bat at the other and the other will respond in kind. |
|---|---|

| For your baby | If you are pregnant with twins, your doctor or midwife may place special emphasis on the amount of weight you gain over the next 4 to 5 weeks. Here's why: If you gain at least 2 pounds by your 24th week (LMP) of pregnancy, you reduce the likelihood of preterm labor. |
|---|---|

| Your body today | Being pregnant with twins is hard work and often means carrying around extra weight and added worries about preterm labor. If you feel exhausted by the end of most days, you are not alone. |
|---|---|

| For your body | Moms with twins should expect to slow down at this stage of the pregnancy. Your midwife or doctor may recommend against aerobic, weight-training or resistance exercise until after you deliver the baby. |
|---|---|

*How I Feel* _____

_____

*My Thoughts* _____

_____

## Day 150    Date _____

| Your baby today | Your baby can easily reach his hand to his mouth today. Gravity, plus the added complication of seeing his own hand, will make this task more difficult outside the womb. |
|---|---|

**or your baby**

Don't forget to take monthly photos of your growing belly so you can document your changing form. Paste them in the spaces allotted throughout this journal so you can one day show your child how deeply connected you were.

**our body today**

You may feel pain, numbness or a tingling sensation in your hip or thigh today. Most likely it's caused by your enlarged uterus putting pressure on the nerves between your legs and your spinal cord.

**or your body**

This may be a persistent feeling as your pregnancy progresses. To ease your discomfort, try changing positions or crouching on your forearms and knees until the feeling subsides.

How I Feel _____

My Thoughts _____

# Day 149    Date _____

**our baby today**

A slippery white substance called vernix is beginning to coat your baby's entire body. This greasy layer helps protect her sensitive skin from being immersed in water for another 148 days.

**or your baby**

Some women opt to labor and even deliver their baby in a tub of warm water. Those who choose a water birth often believe that it eases the baby's transition to the outside world. If you plan on delivering in a hospital, find out if tubs or Jacuzzis are available for this purpose.

**our body today**

If you're a true coffee lover, you may be struggling to cut down on your caffeine intake today.

**or your body**

Try trading your morning coffee for a morning smoothie complete with nonfat yogurt and your favorite blended fruits. The fructose and lactose should provide a lasting shot of energy to power you through the morning.

How I Feel _____

My Thoughts _____

# Day 148    Date _____

**Your baby today**    Your baby girl or boy is starting to get nipples. He or she weighs about 7 ounces and is ove[r] 6 inches long from head to rump.

*For your baby*    The amount of weight your baby gains going forward depends on what you are eating now[,] but it's also determined by how you have eaten throughout your life. Since you can't chang[e] how you've eaten in the past, concentrate on eating healthy today.

**Your body today**    Discomfort due to persistent constipation may make you bloated or uncomfortable today.

*For your body*    Eat some extra fiber today to help speed up your digestion. Add a baked potato (skin on) or [a] pear to your next meal. A glass of orange juice and plenty of water should also be on today[']s menu to help you process the fiber.

How I Feel _____

My Thoughts _____

_____

_____

# Day 147    Date _____

**Your baby today**    Your baby's skin is thickening and is now made up of four layers. Because pigmentation [of] the skin hasn't yet occurred, all babies have the same skin color at this age.

*For your baby*    While most over-the-counter antacids are safe to take during pregnancy, a few of the[m] contain aspirin, which is a pregnancy "don't." Check the ingredients before you buy antacid[s] or check with your doctor or midwife.

**Your body today**    You may feel a bit absent-minded or distracted today as you go about your work or dai[ly] business. Forget where you parked your car? Can't remember your login password? Feelin[g] spacey and unable to focus?

*For your body*    While there's no clear medical explanation, many women claim to have "pregnancy brain[,]" experiences like these all through their pregnancy. If you find that you are distracte[d] by thoughts about your baby or are unusually forgetful and spacey, don't be too har[d] on yourself. This is natural when you're going through so many physical and emotion[al] changes. Use lots of sticky notes and written reminders to make sure the important thing[s] don't get overlooked.

How I Feel _____

_____

_____

My Thoughts _____

Because I had a lot of complications with my pregnancy, it was hard balancing work with trying to keep my mind off what was going on inside my belly.

**—Jennifer D., mother of 2-month-old Lauren**

## Day 146    Date _____

**our baby today**

The nerve cells that control your baby's five senses are developing in their respective areas of the brain.

**or your baby**

Now there are more ways to supply your baby with those brain-building omega-3 fatty acids. The next time you do your groceries, look for omega-3 enhanced foods like salad dressings, cereals, spreads, and sauces as well as omega-3 enriched eggs and meats.

**our body today**

Pressure to name your baby after a family member or unfavorable reactions to your favorite names can add even more stress to the difficult baby-naming process. For those reasons and more, many pregnant women and their partners opt to keep their list of potential baby names a secret. If you can't or don't want to keep your naming process a secret, develop a thick skin for criticism to avoid letting others influence your decision.

**or your body**

Light some candles in your bathroom tonight and enjoy soaking and relaxing in a warm bath. With some peace and quiet and a clear mind, you may be able to feel your baby's movements more easily.

How I Feel _____

My Thoughts _____

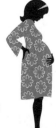

Week 18 Weigh-in:_____lbs

# Day 145　Date _____

**Your baby today**
A doctor can now hear your baby's heartbeat with just a stethoscope.

*For your baby*
This is a great time to "try out" different names on your baby while he or she is still in the womb. Even if you don't know the gender, referring to your baby by a name or term of endearment can help you begin to bond. It can also give you a sense of whether a potential name has the right feel when spoken out loud.

**Your body today**
You may feel the extra work that your heart is doing to pump an extra volume of blood through your body today. If you feel like it's beating harder than ever, it probably is.

*For your body*
If you get a heart-pounding sensation after climbing a set of stairs or exercising, remember to slow down and let your body catch up. These sudden changes in your heartbeat may become more noticeable now and will probably continue until the end of your pregnancy. The good news is, your heart rate will return to normal after you give birth.

How I Feel _____
_____
_____

My Thoughts _____
_____
_____
_____

# Day 144　Date _____

**Your baby today**
Your baby's memory is becoming more sophisticated today.

*For your baby*
Rigorous or high-speed activities that cause you to bounce around a lot (like horseback riding, amusement park rides, skiing, etc) could cause the placenta to separate from the wall of the uterus. This is referred to as placental abruption, an event that can be detrimental to your health and the health of your baby.

**Your body today**
You may notice some extra soreness in your legs and feet today, especially if you stand for long periods of time.

*For your body*
Now may be the time to pack up those high-heeled shoes and make way for flats and casual footwear.

How I Feel _____
_____

## Day 143    Date _____

**our baby today**

Though her eyelids are closed, your baby's eyes move back and forth under the lids. She is now able to sense changes in light.

**or your baby**

Because you're still not used to your protruding belly, you may find that you misjudge your circumference and occasionally bump your "bump" into tables, furniture, and people. While extreme impact (as in a car crash or a fall) could hurt your baby, take solace in the fact that your baby's watery and cushioned environment protects him from minor collisions like these.

**our body today**

If you place a hand at the same level as your belly button, you may be able to feel the top of your uterus.

**or your body**

Stay in tune with your changing body. Because your skin may be dry from stretching to make room for the baby, a daily application of skin lotion in front of the mirror may be the perfect opportunity to take stock of any new changes. You may find that you gain new respect for your body as you watch it transform into a complicated baby-support machine.

*How I Feel* _____

*My Thoughts* _____

## Day 142    Date _____

**our baby today**

Your baby may already show signs of a preference for using his right or left hand.

**or your baby**

You need at least 30 mg of iron today to help your baby produce all the hemoglobin she needs. Pork is a great source of iron, so consider feasting on spaghetti and pork sausage or pork chops and veggies tonight.

**our body today**

If you started your pregnancy at a normal weight, you may be about 9 pounds heavier today. By this point, some women begin to question whether their partner is still attracted to their pregnant figure.

*For your body*

The best thing you can do for your self confidence and your sexual relationship is to spea[k] honestly to your partner. Ask him how he feels about the changes happening to you[r] body. Men react differently to the pregnant form: Some think it's a turn on while others ar[e] intimidated. Once you understand how your partner perceives you and why, you will b[e] better equipped to maintain a healthy sex life throughout the rest of your pregnancy.

*How I Feel* _____

_____

_____

*My Thoughts* _____

_____

_____

_____

# Day 141    Date _____

## Your baby today

Your baby has just enough room to float comfortably in the amniotic sac and mov[e] as she pleases.

*For your baby*

While some facilities now offer sonograms to pregnant women for the sole benefit [of] providing a new picture of their unborn baby, the American Pregnancy Association warn[s] against such a practice. You should only get a sonogram when it's recommended by you[r] own physician and performed by licensed medical professionals.

## Your body today

If you've ever had breast enhancement or reduction surgery, you may be wondering [if] breastfeeding is out of the question.

*For your body*

Many women who have undergone breast surgery, especially breast enlargement or surge[ry] to remove lumps, can still breastfeed their child. Talk to your surgeon and your medic[al] provider to discuss the details of your surgery and find out if you are still likely to have ful[ly] functioning milk ducts.

*How I Feel* _____

_____

_____

*My Thoughts* _____

_____

_____

_____

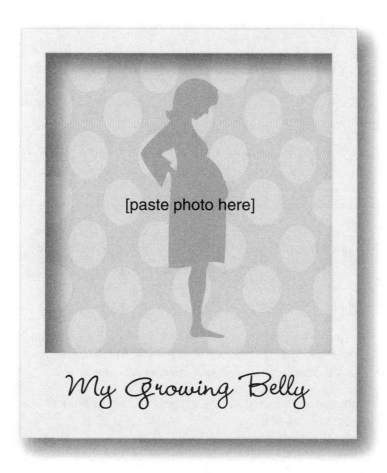

[paste photo here]

*My Growing Belly*

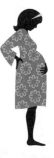

# Day 140    Date _____

**Your baby today**

Your baby has reached a milestone. She will no longer be measured from the crown of h head to her rump. She is now measured from head to heel! If you were to measure h today, she would be over 8 ½ inches long.

*For your baby*

Sharing your thoughts and feelings in this journal is one of the best ways to commemora this amazing time in your life and share it with your child. One day, years from now, you ca sit down together and read your entries. If you don't have something to say every day, k sure to record your hopes and dreams for your baby when the mood strikes. It's one of th greatest gifts you can offer her.

**Your body today**

If you are small-breasted, even in pregnancy, you may wonder whether you'll be able produce enough milk for your baby.

*For your body*

Rest assured that breast size is unrelated to milk production. The amount of milk you ca produce for your baby is influenced by your overall health and whether your breasts a properly stimulated.

*How I Feel* _____

_____

_____

*My Thoughts* _____

_____

_____

# Day 139    Date _____

**Your baby today**

Your baby's eyelids have finished developing today.

*For your baby*

Because newborns are still developing their coordination, they can scratch their ti fingernails against their face and eyes. A pair of cotton baby mittens, sold at most ba apparel stores, can protect your newborn from his own unruly hand movements.

**Your body today**

You may find yourself craving the intimacy of sex but feel uncomfortable or unsatisfied your usual sex positions.

*For your body*

Just as you are learning to sleep comfortably on your side, you will be a happier and mo satisfied pregnant woman if you can learn to enjoy sex in the side-by-side position. spooning doesn't do the trick, you may want to try straddling your partner while he's on h back or while he's sitting on a chair.

# Day 138   Date _____

**our baby today**

Your baby is swallowing more amniotic fluid now, allowing her new digestive system to practice absorbing the water. Her kidneys are removing some of the waste, but she still needs your kidneys to do most of the work.

**or your baby**

Now that your baby is relying on your kidneys, keep them healthy and free of infection. Stick to cotton underwear and loose pants, drinks lots of water and unsweetened cranberry juice, and urinate before and after you have sex.

**our body today**

You are suddenly aware of your baby's subtle movements and it's adding a whole new level of excitement to your pregnancy. You may even start to notice that your baby has a schedule. He may kick more after meals or late at night.

**or your body**

Enjoy the novelty of feeling your baby first-hand. It is one of the truly amazing miracles of pregnancy, one that helps foster a strong connection between mother and child. If you think of this activity as a form of communication, you can begin to interpret changes in his behavior. That strong poke or that series of twitches may indicate irritability in response to a loud noise, excitement about something you just ate, or a desire for you to roll over to your other side.

How I Feel

My Thoughts

Week 19 Weigh-in:____lbs

## Day 137   Date _____

**Your baby today**

The growth of your baby's head is slowing down and the growth of his body picking up considerably.

**For your baby**

Your baby's bones are a big part of his growth and development this month. Because yo baby will pull from your own supply of calcium if he's not getting enough, it's a good idea fill up on calcium-rich foods and meet your daily calcium requirement of 1,000 mg. Navy pinto beans are both generous sources of calcium.

**Your body today**

You may have some ideas for how you want your labor and delivery to play out. Wome often work with their midwife or OB/GYN to develop a birth plan that expresses their goa (a natural birth versus a Caesarean, etc.) and their preferences (whether they want breastfeed or bottle-feed, etc.).

**For your body**

Start writing down your desires for the day you deliver. Important things to consider ar whether you want pain medication and if so, what kind; whether you want to breastfeed; ar who you want in the delivery room. Your opinions may change over the next 136 days aft talking to other moms and researching your options, but this will at least get you thinkir about the right things. Note of caution: don't be fooled into thinking that you can actua plan everything about your birth. While your medical team will take your preferences in consideration, Mother Nature will almost always throw a curveball on the day you deliver.

*How I Feel* _____

_____

*My Thoughts* _____

_____

## Day 136   Date _____

**Your baby today**

Your baby weighs about 12 ounces today, the same as a can of soup.

**For your baby**

While most women don't need a medical reason to steer clear of reptiles, the CE recommends removing them from your home and keeping a safe distance from all reptil during pregnancy. Up to 90 percent of these animals carry salmonella bacteria. One particul kind of salmonella bacteria can cross the placenta and cause miscarriage, stillbirth, ar preterm labor.

**Your body today**

If you're pregnant with multiples, you may find that first trimester morning sickness h given way to second trimester fits of hunger. You may feel like there's no end to the amou of food you could eat today.

or your body

Listen to those hunger pangs to ensure that you are gaining enough weight. Try to eat at least three meals and four to five hefty snacks per day to keep up with your body's needs. Eating something at least every two hours is recommended at this stage of pregnancy.

How I Feel

My Thoughts

## Day 135  Date _____

our baby today

No matter what kind of hair your baby will have at birth, right now it is completely white and very short.

or your baby

If you want to give your baby the calcium he or she needs but you suffer from lactose intolerance, there are plenty of alternative calcium sources to meet your needs. Non-dairy foods that are high in calcium include sardines with bones, canned salmon with bones, tofu (if it's processed with calcium sulfate), calcium-fortified soy milk or orange juice, and green, leafy vegetables.

our body today

Not sure how your body will perform under the physical rigors of labor? Make sure you have the right people there to support you in the delivery room. Consider hiring a doula, whose job is to keep you relaxed and focused throughout the entire labor and delivery process.

or your body

If you think you may need the kind of support that a doula provides, start searching for one now. Seek referrals from medical specialists, family members, or friends. Keep in mind that you will probably need to hire a labor assistant with your own money, as most health insurance policies will not cover the cost.

How I Feel

My Thoughts

—Jin, mother of 9-month-old Ming

# Day 134　Date _____

**Your baby today**

Your baby's skin is full of tiny wrinkles that will disappear once she develops a the fat she needs.

*For your baby*

Being underweight in pregnancy can starve your baby of nutrients that are crucial to h growth. If you are not gaining as much weight as you should, try these higher-calor substitutions: switch from skim milk to whole milk, exchange that vegetable oil spread f real butter, and enjoy healthy, high-fat foods like salmon and red meat.

**Your body today**

This is a difficult time for many women when it comes to body image. You may be so use to resisting weight gain that it may be difficult to embrace the idea of putting on 25 to extra pounds. Remind yourself that this is one of the first sacrifices you will make for yo child and that exercise and healthy eating will help you return to your previous weight aft delivery.

*For your body*

If you're going to indulge in sweet snacks today, opt for sweets with some nutritional bene like ice cream and milk shakes for a calcium boost, or oatmeal cookies for a healthy dose fiber.

*How I Feel* _____

_____

_____

*My Thoughts* _____

_____

_____

# Day 133    Date _____

**Your baby today**

Your baby has just reached the halfway mark in her development! If you pat your belly right now, you might be able to wake her up to congratulate her.

**For your baby**

You have done a great job guiding your little one safely through the first half of her life in the womb. What you've already learned about your child and about pregnancy over the last 133 days will help steer you through the next 133 days with more confidence. The best thing you can do for your baby going forward is to trust your motherly instincts, because they are getting sharper and sharper every day.

**Your body today**

Congratulations! You've made it halfway through your pregnancy. The countdown continues, but you're well on your way to having your new son or daughter. Don't beat yourself up over things you can't change: that glass of wine you had before you knew you were pregnant, that French fry habit you developed in the first trimester, the day you used chemical cleaners or painted a wall of the nursery. Instead, congratulate yourself on all the sacrifices you have already made for your child and think of how far you have come and how much you have learned about yourself, your body, and your baby.

**For your body**

Now is a good time to decide which childbirth classes you would like to attend. Your local hospital, community center, or doctor's office will sponsor courses on topics including labor breathing techniques, hypnobirthing, breastfeeding, and infant CPR. Register for the classes of your choice and recruit your partner to accompany you to some, if not all, of them.

How I Feel .............................................................................................................................

My Thoughts .............................................................................................................................

# Day 132    Date _____

**Your baby today**

Your baby is about 10 inches long now and weighs close to 14 ounces.

**For your baby**

Put aside some time today for daddy-baby bonding. Encourage your partner to sit with his hand on your belly to feel the baby's movements. Let him know that she can now hear his voice if he wants to talk to her. If he's too embarrassed to talk to the baby, suggest that he read her a story so she gets more familiar with the sound of his voice.

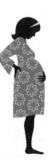

Week 20 Weigh-in: _____ lbs

| Your body today | One more month and you will have made it to your third and final trimester! You should b gaining about a pound a week at this point. |
|---|---|
| *For your body* | Make yourself a fruit salad for snacking between meals. You'll get a wide variety of vitami (including A and C) and nutrients (including potassium and fiber) while satisfying yo sweet tooth. |

How I Feel _____

_____

_____

My Thoughts _____

_____

_____

_____

# Day 131　　Date _____

| Your baby today | Your baby's skin has taken on a reddish hue today. It's also thicker and less transparent. |
|---|---|
| *For your baby* | If you have other children, get them ready for the new baby's arrival and invite them become involved with anything related to the baby. For example, let them help you decora the nursery, pick out baby gear, or hear the heartbeat at your next doctor's appointmer Making a big deal out of their upcoming status as "big brother" or "big sister" may also ea their anxieties about sharing your attention with another child. |
| Your body today | Lying on your back now feels fairly uncomfortable. This is nature's way of telling you change position. |
| *For your body* | After 20 weeks of pregnancy, avoid lying on your back for an extended period of time as could stop blood from flowing to your baby. This will not only change the way you sleep, b it may also change how you exercise. |

How I Feel _____

_____

_____

My Thoughts _____

_____

_____

_____

**our baby today**

The part of your baby's brain that produces brain cells is now maturing at a rapid rate.

**or your baby**

If you are trying to save money on baby gear and furniture but you can't get that gorgeous but expensive sleigh crib out of your mind, consider purchasing a gently used version on Ebay or Craigslist.

**our body today**

Now that your pregnancy is out in the open and you're showing, you may feel as though your boss or coworkers treat you differently. You may resent getting too much attention for your pregnant condition and not enough attention for the work you're doing. You may also be concerned that your coworkers no longer take you as seriously because they assume that you're preoccupied by your physical condition.

**or your body**

These are common concerns for pregnant women in the workplace. While some of these issues are best handled by discussing your concerns with your boss or coworkers, don't be afraid to take action if you are a victim of pregnancy discrimination. You are protected from such treatment under the Pregnancy Discrimination Act (PDA) which makes it illegal for your boss to hire, fire, or refuse to promote you based on the fact that you're pregnant. To read more about how you're protected from pregnancy discrimination, go to http://www.eeoc.gov/types/pregnancy.html.

How I Feel _____

_____

My Thoughts _____

_____

_____

**our baby today**

Your baby's pancreas is on its way to becoming a functioning organ.

**or your baby**

Start registering for baby items today with the help of a friend, family member, or—better yet—an experienced mom. While registering in the store allows you to closely evaluate the look and feel of products like swings, high chairs, and bedding, registering online may be less overwhelming and often allows you instant access to customer ratings and reviews. You may find that a mix of online and offline shopping is the best approach.

**our body today**

An increase in estrogen levels is increasing blood flow to your breasts and vagina. As a result, you may feel more aroused than usual lately.

*For your body*

Take advantage of this boost in your libido to try out some new pregnancy-friendly se
positions. With a little determination, and a lot of well-placed pillows, you can still mak
a lot of them work at this stage. Avoid positions where you need to lay flat on your back i
favor of rear-entry positions that keep pressure off your belly.

How I Feel _____

_____

My Thoughts _____

_____

## Day 128 Date _____

**Your baby today**

Today your baby has working sweat glands, fully formed fingernails, and distinct lips.

*For your baby*

Take a close look at your family budget today and see if there is something you can cut o
of the budget to allow for added spending on diapers, formula, clothing, and other gea
One thing that may be easy to cut from the budget is the expense of eating out. Having
newborn will automatically make you more likely to dine in the comfort of your own home

**Your body today**

After a close review of your budget, you may need the stress release that exercise provide

*For your body*

If you feel frustrated at home or at work, taking a long walk, playing a prenatal exercise DV
at home, or going for a swim may leave you feeling renewed. Eating complex carbohydrate
about an hour before exercising can help supply you with the energy you'll need. Mix u
and enjoy a small bowl of whole-wheat pasta salad or half a wheat bagel with cream chees
before heading to your workout.

How I Feel _____

_____

My Thoughts _____

_____

## Day 127 Date _____

**Your baby today**

If your baby is a boy, his testes are making their way down from his pelvis to his scrotum.
your baby is a girl, her vagina is beginning to take shape.

*For your baby*

Get ready for diaper changes! Special care must be taken depending on your baby's gende
Girls should always be wiped from front to back to prevent infection. If you have a boy, cov

his penis with an absorbent cloth as soon as it's exposed to the air. Otherwise, you risk being sprayed. Clean all around the scrotum and make sure the penis is pointing down before securing the new diaper. (A penis that points up will cause constant diaper leaks.) Feel like an expert? Soon you will be.

**our body today**

While it's still early in your pregnancy, your mind may be racing about what will happen on the day you deliver the baby. You may wonder what a labor pain really feels like and whether you'll be able to endure it. You may be concerned that the baby will come quickly and you won't make it to the hospital in time.

**or your body**

Rest assured that the average first-time labor lasts about 15 hours, which is plenty of time to get to the hospital or birth center. If you think that it may ease your worries, make a few practice runs to and from your destination to familiarize yourself with the best and fastest route. Designate a neighbor or family member to help you out in the off chance that your partner is out of reach or traveling and can't drive you there himself.

How I Feel ........................................................................................................................................

........................................................................................................................................

My Thoughts ........................................................................................................................................

........................................................................................................................................

---

# Day 126  Date _____

**our baby today**

Your baby is starting to look a lot like he will as a newborn, except that his skin is still slightly transparent.

**or your baby**

It's normal to have more vaginal discharge than usual during pregnancy, but if you notice anything particularly unusual like discharge that's yellow, green, cottage-cheese like, or foul-smelling, don't ignore it. It could be a sign of a kidney or urinary tract infection that, if untreated, could lead to preterm labor.

**our body today**

By now you are probably used to giving a urine sample at the start of each doctor's visit. You will probably have no trouble providing this sample, as your uterus is positioned directly above your bladder and the constant urge to urinate has returned.

**or your body**

When you hand over that urine sample, you are providing for early detection of three different kinds of complications. Bacteria in the urine could indicate a kidney or urinary tract infection. Protein might also indicate an infection or it could be an indicator of preeclampsia. Sugar in the urine is a red flag for gestational diabetes. To make sure warning signs of these complications don't go unnoticed, mark all your medical appointments on your calendar and don't miss a visit.

Week 21 Weigh-in:_____lbs

*How I Feel* _____

*My Thoughts* _____

## Day 125  Date _____

| | |
|---|---|
| Your baby today | Your baby now has a mouth full of (permanent) tooth buds beneath her gums. |
| *For your baby* | It may be too early to buy your baby a toothbrush, but it's safe to say that you'll soon need teething ring and some numbing ointment for her sore gums. |
| Your body today | If you are a vegetarian, you may have a difficult time meeting the daily iron requirement c 30 mg. |
| *For your body* | As a vegetarian, you need every bit of iron you can get from the greens you eat. For tha reason, avoid eating them with tea or coffee or shortly before or after taking antacids. A of these things can impede your body's ability to absorb iron. Vitamin C, on the other han facilitates iron absorption. Add a glass of O.J. to your iron-rich meals to soak in more iron. |

*How I Feel* _____

*My Thoughts* _____

## Day 124  Date _____

| | |
|---|---|
| Your baby today | The fine hair that covers your baby's body has just grown darker in color. |
| *For your baby* | Start thinking about where your baby will sleep when he comes home from the hospita Many babies spend their first weeks and months at their parents' bedside in a bassinet c co-sleeper (a raised baby bed that attaches securely alongside your own mattress). Som sleep right in bed with their parents. Since most parents choose to have their newborn clos by for breastfeeding convenience and peace of mind, make sure you have what you need provide that option. |
| Your body today | You may find that you are exhausted by the end of the day, but still have troubl getting to sleep. |

or your body | Try taking a warm bath or shower before bed to relax your muscles and ease your stress. Reconfigure your pillows to support your belly and back. If your partner is willing, a shoulder, back, or leg massage right before bed is sometimes the fastest route to deep sleep.

How I Feel _____

My Thoughts _____

## Day 123    Date _____

Your baby today | Now that your baby's inner ear bones have hardened, she can hear a whole lot better.

or your baby | While there are no clear findings that it boosts their intelligence, playing classical music to your unborn baby can certainly do no harm. It may not influence his long-term academic success, but it will probably soothe and relax both of you in the short term.

Your body today | When you spit after brushing, you may see a little blood. You may even notice little bumps on your gums (pyogenic granulomas) that are highly sensitive and apt to bleed when brushed.

or your body | Pregnancy hormones can cause your gums to be more sensitive and swollen, thus more apt to bleed. Frequent brushing and flossing will help make your gums stronger and healthier. Eat and drink foods rich in vitamin C to help keep gingivitis at bay and support the repair of healthy gum tissue.

How I Feel _____

My Thoughts _____

## Day 122    Date _____

Your baby today | Your baby's eyes are well developed, but his irises are still lacking in color.

or your baby | There is no need to avoid your microwave oven during pregnancy. While high amounts of radiation could do damage to fetal tissue, the small amount of radiation given off by your microwave is unlikely to have any effect on your tissue or your baby's.

Your body today | Look down at your belly. Is there a thin white or dark line running from your belly button down to your pelvic area? If so, this is called the linea negra.

*For your body*   No one is quite sure why this line forms, but it will go away a few months after the baby i delivered. It is one of the more elegant skin irregularities of pregnancy and may actuall warrant a photograph for the scrapbook.

*How I Feel* _____

*My Thoughts* _____

_____

## Day 121   Date _____

Your baby today   Your baby can hear how your voice changes when you get excited or angry. He will know th rhythm and variations in your voice well by the time he is a newborn.

*For your baby*   Use gloves and open the closest window for proper ventilation when using chemica household cleaning products. There isn't a lot of research regarding the potential effec of these products on your unborn child, but most are thought to be safe if direct contact avoided and if the area is properly ventilated. If you would rather be on the safe side, han over some of your cleaning duties to your partner or switch to some of the new "greer products on the market. You can even make a safe, homemade cleaning solution with a m of vinegar, baking soda, and salt.

Your body today   You may notice that your face is oilier than usual today, a typical side effect of pregnancy.

*For your body*   Invest in a pack of blotting papers to cut down on excess facial oil during the day. Wash you face twice a day with nothing but soap for sensitive skin and water.

*How I Feel* _____

*My Thoughts* _____

_____

## Day 120   Date _____

Your baby today   Your baby is developing more blood vessels in her lungs to prepare for her first gulp of ai

*For your baby*   If you're having trouble setting up your baby's nursery so it looks and feels just right, let th ancient Chinese principles of feng shui guide you. Place the crib so that your baby can se you when you walk in the room. Consider using lots of white in the room, as that is the col of creativity. To enhance energy flow, leave a fan blowing on a low setting, hang a mobi near an open window, or play gentle music.

**our body today**

Leaking urine every time you cough, sneeze, or laugh may be a consistent problem at this stage of your pregnancy.

**or your body**

If you don't want to be caught off-guard by this common pregnancy nuisance, consider wearing pantyliners.

*How I Feel* _____

_____

*My Thoughts* _____

_____

# Day 119 Date _____

**our baby today**

Your baby has grown to be about a foot long! He now weighs 1¼ to 1½ pounds, about as much as a jar of pickles.

**or your baby**

It may be time to speak with your rabbi, priest, or officiant about planning a ceremony to initiate your baby into the community. Whether it's a brit malah, brit bat, or christening, religious tradition may require that the ceremony be held as early as a week after birth. You'll be in no condition to handle the planning right after your baby is born, so do as much as you can in advance.

**our body today**

You may be embarrassed to find that you are passing more gas than usual these days. Pregnancy-related indigestion can also leave you feeling bloated and prone to burping spells.

**or your body**

Most pregnant women have problems with gas and indigestion in the second trimester and beyond. It is one of the quirks of pregnancy that you may have to grin and bear. Exercising and avoiding gas-inducing foods like beans, fried or greasy foods, and broccoli may offer some relief.

*How I Feel* _____

_____

*My Thoughts* _____

_____

Week 22 Weigh-in:_____lbs

# Day 118    Date _____

**Your baby today**

Air sacs have developed in your baby's developing lungs, but those sacs will remain deflate until air enters.

*For your baby*

Essential amino acids are those that your body cannot produce on its own. To help you baby get the essential amino acids she needs to build healthy tissue and organs, it's bes to eat a variety of "complete proteins." These include meat, fish, poultry, eggs, and dair products.

**Your body today**

You can probably see and feel that your breasts and uterus are continuing to grow an stretch as your pregnancy progresses. The top of your uterus can now be felt a few inche above your belly button.

*For your body*

Eating 2–3 servings of red meat, poultry, or fish today will help support the growth of you breast and uterine tissue.

How I Feel _____

_____

_____

My Thoughts _____

_____

_____

_____

# Day 117    Date _____

**Your baby today**

If your baby were born today, there is a 40–50 percent chance that she would survive wit expert care. In another month, that percentage will increase to about 80 percent. Re assured, though, that premature births this early are very, very rare, and your doctor woul likely be able to stop your labor if it did begin now. Be sure to call your medical profession if you experience amniotic fluid leakage, spotting, or contractions.

*For your baby*

If you are one of the 2 to 5 percent of women who develop gestational (pregnancy-relatec diabetes, you'll need to adhere to a strict diet and exercise plan to reduce the effect on you baby. Babies born to women with gestational diabetes may be too large to fit through th birth canal. They may also have breathing problems, jaundice, and other health issues.

**Your body today**

You may be asked to take a glucose screening test at your next medical appointment. You be given a very sugary mixture to drink and your blood will be drawn about an hour later check the amount of sugar that remains in your blood.

or your body

While the sickly sweet mixture you're asked to drink may seem like a form of punishment, keep in mind that a glucose screening test could be the key to diagnosing gestational diabetes before it leads to health problems for you and your baby. A positive glucose screening test does not necessarily mean that you have gestational diabetes, but it does warrant further testing.

How I Feel

My Thoughts

# Day 116     Date _____

our baby today

Surfactant, a key substance that helps the lungs expand at birth, is now in production in your baby's body.

or your baby

Have some fun using your baby's due date to get to know him or her. Find out which zodiac sign your child will have, which qualities are attributed to that sign, and how it interacts with your own.

our body today

A bout of cramps or Braxton Hicks contractions may have you worried about preterm labor today.

or your body

Only about 12 percent of babies in the U.S. are born before 37 weeks, and many of them are intentionally induced for health reasons. Regardless, it doesn't hurt to learn the signs of preterm labor: an increase in vaginal discharge, discharge that is suddenly watery, mucus-like, or bloody, vaginal bleeding or spotting, stomach pain, cramps, or more than four contractions per hour, pelvic pressure that feels like your baby is descending, and lower back pain (especially if you haven't had it before). Play it safe and call your doctor or midwife if you aren't sure whether what you're feeling is preterm labor.

How I Feel

My Thoughts

Your baby today

Your baby is still very slender, but she's beginning to gain more and more fat and her face i filling out as a result.

For your baby

The American Medical Association cautions against standing for more than four hours at time after 24 weeks (LMP) of pregnancy. They also advise against standing for more tha thirty minutes after 32 weeks. Doing so may increase your risk of preterm contractions an labor. If your job requires you to stand for long periods of time, you may want to request change in your job responsibilities.

Your body today

If you haven't found out whether you're having a boy or a girl, you'll discover that everyone you know—and even some you don't—are convinced they can predict which you're having You may even have your own conviction about the sex of your child.

For your body

See if common lore predicts a boy or a girl in your future: If you crave sweets and if your baby heart rate is 150 or above, traditional wisdom says you're carrying a girl. If you crave salt foods and meat, and if your baby's heart rate is closer to 140, you may be carrying a boy.

How I Feel _____

_____

_____

My Thoughts _____

_____

_____

Your baby today

The skin on your baby's hands and feet is now thicker than the skin on the rest of hi growing body.

For your baby

Having a newborn means worrying over every irregular breath, skin rash, bowel movemen (or lack thereof), and crying spell. Invest in an infant health guide that you can consu during these inevitable, middle-of-the-night panic sessions. Your pediatrician is always th best adviser, but having an objective, expert resource at arm's length will help you determin when to call the doctor and when to go back to sleep. A great resource is *The America Academy of Pediatrics Caring for Your Baby and Young Child.*

Your body today

By now you may have formed ideas about the kind of labor and birth you want. It may be natural birth free of any pain medications, a pain-managed birth where the epidural come to your aid as soon as you need it, or a home birth assisted by your midwife and doula.

*or your body*

No matter what your preferences dictate, you will greatly benefit by planning for the unplanned. These days, about one in three women deliver their babies by C-section. Even if a C-section is the last thing you want or imagine for yourself, do yourself a favor by reading up on surgical birth. Being informed will help ease your concerns if your labor does end in a C-section.

*How I Feel*

*My Thoughts*

> With my planned C-section, I loved knowing the exact date the baby was going to arrive and anticipating the minute he would be here when we were in the operating room. I didn't like the fact that the nurses were constantly in and out of the room day after day, monitoring this and that and looking at the incision. I just wanted time alone to stare at my new baby!
>
> —Paige B., mother of 6-month-old Ian

## Day 113 Date _____

**our baby today**

Your baby's days and nights are set to the symphony of your voice, heartbeat, and stomach gurgles.

*or your baby*

It's important to get enough rest at regular times. This may help your baby be better able to tell the difference between night and day after he's born (but don't count on it!).

**our body today**

Your doctor or midwife has probably started to measure your fundal height (the distance from the top of your uterus to your pubic bone) at every appointment. This will help her measure the growth of your baby. It may also tell her something about the baby's position in the uterus.

*For your body*

If you want to know whether your fundal height is in the normal range, it should be roughly equivalent to the number of weeks you've been pregnant. If it's been 20 weeks since your last menstrual cycle, your fundal height should be in the 18-22 cm range. Measuring large or small for your gestational age is not always a matter of concern. It may just mean that your due date is off, your baby is on the larger side, or your muscles are more stretched out.

*How I Feel*

*My Thoughts*

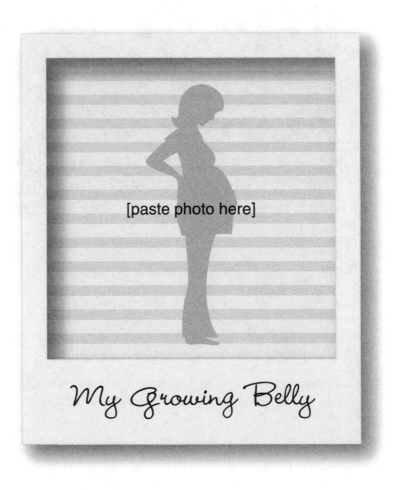

My Growing Belly

# Day 112    Date _____

**Your baby today**

Your baby's nostrils are beginning to open now. Pretty soon his eyes will open as well.

**For your baby**

If you plan on working after the baby comes and you've been putting off your daycare search, now's the time to get back on track. You have a better chance of getting your child into the daycare of your dreams if you reserve a spot early. Later on you might change your mind and decide to stay home with the baby or you may find a nanny or a daycare closer to home. But for now, you (and your boss) will have peace of mind knowing that there's a solid plan in place for when you return to work.

**Your body today**

Your face and eyelids may have seemed puffy and swollen when you woke up this morning. During pregnancy, the extra fluid in your body can collect beneath the thin tissue in your face.

**For your body**

As the day progresses and gravity has its way, facial swelling will go down on its own. A cool compress may speed things along.

How I Feel _____

_____

My Thoughts _____

_____

_____

# Day 111    Date _____

**Your baby today**

The nerves around your baby's lips have recently grown more sensitive. Some experts think this helps her find your nipple for proper breastfeeding.

**For your baby**

Breastfeeding may be natural, but it doesn't come naturally for all women and babies. Many women struggle to get their baby to latch on properly. A proper latch can mean more comfort for mom and more milk for baby. Find out if your hospital or birth center employs onsite lactation consultants to help you as you learn to breastfeed.

**Your body today**

Your breasts are now preparing for the job of feeding your baby. Not only are your nipples larger and darker in color (like two giant bull's-eyes for her mouth), but you may also notice that they are leaking an early form of breast milk called colostrum.

Week 23 Weigh-in:_____lbs

*For your body*

If you plan on breastfeeding, take time to read up on proper latch techniques and breastfeeding positions. You may even want to consider purchasing a breast pump ahead of time. Some health insurance policies will reimburse you for the full expense, so check to see if that's the case with yours. You may also be able to rent a hospital-grade pump to take home with you from the hospital.

*How I Feel* _____

_____

_____

*My Thoughts* _____

_____

_____

# Day 110    Date _____

Your baby today

Your baby has a strong umbilical cord that extends about 22 inches long. This thick cord made up of two arteries and a vein, is the key to your baby's survival.

*For your baby*

Unless you always have a babysitter handy, your choice of restaurants will soon become more limited. Keep an eye open for kid-friendly restaurants in your local area. Don't assume that fast-food joints and chain restaurants are your only option. Many coffee shops, delis and family-owned restaurants are natural gathering spots for people with young children.

Your body today

Lower back aches may now plague you at the end of a long day.

*For your body*

Because your posture during pregnancy tends to compensate for the added weight up front, you may need to take measures to prevent lower backache. If you are standing for a long period of time, try putting one foot up on a stepstool or box to take some pressure off of your back. If your mattress is on the soft side, insert a piece of plywood between the mattress and the box spring. Severe back pain during pregnancy is not the norm, and may be a sign of kidney infection or preterm labor. Alert your doctor if the pain is very strong and persistent.

*How I Feel* _____

_____

_____

*My Thoughts* _____

_____

_____

**Your baby today**   Your baby's brain now has a billion neurons—all he will need for his lifetime.

**For your baby**   If you haven't finished registering for baby gear, make that your goal this week. The longer you wait, the more likely you are to receive duplicate items or gifts that you just don't need. Afraid to commit to the items you've chosen? Don't worry: you can always add, delete, or return them as needed.

**Your body today**   You may notice that after a day of typing on the computer, you experience tingling or pain in your hands, wrists, and/or lower arms. That's because the tissue in your arms and hands is swelling and putting more pressure on the ligament in your wrist called the "carpal tunnel." Even those who aren't prone to what's called carpal tunnel syndrome may experience it during pregnancy.

**For your body**   Making ergonomic adjustments to your work area can decrease the severity of carpal tunnel. When typing, your arm should bend at a 90-degree angle. Your wrist should be angled slightly downward when you type, not upward. Depending on how much pain you're experiencing, you may want to invest in an ergonomic keyboard, wrist guard, and mouse.

How I Feel _____

_____

My Thoughts _____

_____

_____

**Your baby today**   Your baby now has a more regular exercise routine. Her level of activity probably peaks around midnight.

**For your baby**   While you have every right to satisfy your pregnancy cravings, don't fool yourself into thinking that all pregnancy cravings are your body's way of supplying the nutrients you're lacking. Sometimes an intense desire for a hot fudge sundae is just an intense desire for a hot fudge sundae.

**Your body today**   End-of-day fatigue and pregnancy discomforts may become more persistent as your pregnancy progresses.

**For your body**   Keep the month before and after your due date wide open. While you may be tempted to pencil in that weekend excursion or wedding two weeks before your due date, you will probably want to keep a low profile and relax as Day 1 approaches.

## Day 107    Date _____

**Your baby today**

Before now, your baby's heartbeat stayed fairly steady. Today your baby's heartbeat fluctuate more, sometimes in response to her environment.

*For your baby*

If you like hearing your baby's heartbeat at your medical appointments, you may be happy to know that stores now sell prenatal heartbeat monitors you can use to listen to your baby heartbeat and hiccups at home. This is just one way to bond with the little one growin inside you—pick your favorite (massaging your belly, talking, reading, singing to her, etc and make it a priority today.

**Your body today**

Bending over may begin to feel like a chore as you get closer to the third trimester c pregnancy. Putting on shoes, picking things up off the floor, and grabbing things off th bottom shelf may squish your enlarged belly in an uncomfortable way.

*For your body*

Get in the habit of asking other people for help, because soon it will be a necessity. You find that most people are eager to assist you on the train, at work, in the grocery store, etc If putting on shoes is a problem, consider switching to clogs, mules, or flip-flops so you ca put them on standing up.

As a way to bond with both my children while I was pregnant, I used to sing every song I knew that came on the radio to them when I was driving alone in the car. That way they not only heard my voice, but also got used to my singing, so it was a familiar sound when they arrived.

—Margot C., mother of 6-year-old Isabelle and 3-year-old Jean-Claude

How I Feel _____

My Thoughts _____

## Day 106 Date _____

**Your baby today**

Your baby may be feeling hungry right now. Experts speculate that this is why he drinks in some amniotic fluid.

**For your baby**

It's a good idea to start reading parenting books and talking to other parents about their tricks and tips. You won't have a lot of time for reading once the baby arrives, and you might want to get a jump on developing your own parenting philosophy.

**Your body today**

While some women are still basking in the "honeymoon stage" of pregnancy at this point, others may grow tired of constantly talking about and thinking about their pregnancy. Don't feel guilty if you're having these feelings. Most women crave an escape from pregnancy at some point.

**For your body**

Make a date with friends this week to enjoy a night of dancing, an afternoon of movie-watching, or at the very least—some baby-free conversation. You can also make an agreement with your partner to reserve a day of the week for all things unrelated to the baby. Make a point to talk about your relationship, your day, your career goals, etc. and take comfort in the fact that there's more to you than your baby bump.

How I Feel _____

My Thoughts _____

Week 24 Weigh-in:____lbs

# Day 105 Date _____

### Your baby today

Your baby weighs about 2 pounds today and is starting to get cramped for space insid[ ] your uterus.

### For your baby

Not sure which questions to ask a potential daycare provider? Start with these three: Wha[ ] is the ratio of daycare providers to infants? (Make sure the answer complies with sta[ ] regulations.) What will an average day at daycare be like for my baby? Is it okay if I stop [ ] the daycare unannounced to check in on my child? This last question is very important. B[ ] wary of any daycare that says no.

### Your body today

Swollen hands and fingers may be causing your rings to feel too tight.

### For your body

Before swelling makes this task impossible, run your hands under cold water and rub soa[ ] against your rings until you can slide them off your fingers. Stash them somewhere for sa[ ] keeping until your baby arrives.

How I Feel _____
_____

My Thoughts _____
_____

# Day 104 Date _____

### Your baby today

Your baby can grab hold of his feet today and may even suck on his toes!

### For your baby

One way to keep track of your baby's health this far into your pregnancy is to count his kick[ ] Here's how: Note the time it takes him to complete ten movements. The trick is to do this [ ] approximately the same time each day when your baby tends to be most active. In genera[ ] healthy babies make at least ten movements within two hours, though most do it in les[ ] than 15 minutes. Let your healthcare provider know of any changes in your baby's norm[ ] pattern or if your baby takes more than two hours to complete ten movements.

### Your body today

When you look down today, you may have to bend forward a little to see your feet.

### For your body

Treat yourself to a pedicure while you can still see your feet and appreciate your toes. N[ ] only is it getting harder and harder to bend over and paint your own toes, but a full leg ar[ ] foot massage can help with persistent aches and swelling.

How I Feel _____

## Day 103    Date _____

**Your baby today**

Your baby is already going through the motion of breathing, but since there is no air in the womb this is mostly done to prepare his lungs for birth.

**For your baby**

Don't get stuck in a repetitive eating routine. The more varied your diet, the better the chance that you're supplying your body and your baby's with the wide range of nutrients it needs. Need a new mini-meal idea: how about a tomato-and-Swiss-cheese melt on whole grain pita?

**Your body today**

Whether you've signed up for a Lamaze class or bought yourself a book on hypnobirthing, you're probably wondering how well these pain management techniques will work in the moment.

**For your body**

There's no easy way to predict how your body and mind will handle the rigors of labor. All you can do is have confidence in yourself, prepare yourself mentally for the challenge ahead, and pick up as many coping mechanisms as you can before the big day. Here's one more coping mechanism to add to your arsenal: Create a mix of empowering, invigorating and relaxing songs to take with you to the hospital or to play while laboring at home.

How I Feel _____

My Thoughts _____

## Day 102    Date _____

**Your baby today**

If your partner puts his ear to your belly today, he may be able to hear the baby's heartbeat.

**For your baby**

No one is more excited to meet your child than you and your partner . . . except maybe the baby's grandparents. Try to involve them as much as possible in the preparations leading up to your due date. Ask them what they want the baby to call them. Find out if there are any items they kept from your childhood or your partner's childhood. Adding these items to your baby's nursery is a small gesture, but it may mean a great deal to them.

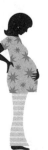

| Your body today | You may be alarmed to find out that the maternity clothes you bought at the beginning your pregnancy no longer fit. The waistbands are uncomfortably tight and the shirts a riding up over your baby bump. |
|---|---|
| *For your body* | If you think you'll have at least one more child or if you've been wearing the same pair pants for a week, it may make sense to stock up on a new crop of maternity clothing. Stick basics that you can wear again and again, plus one or two splurge items that you can we on special occasions. |

How I Feel _____

_____

My Thoughts _____

_____

## Day 101    Date _____

| Your baby today | Your baby responds to both sound and touch today. |
|---|---|
| *For your baby* | If it's your faith or tradition to do so, now is a good time to choose your child's godparen and ask them if they will accept the honor. |
| Your body today | You may be lagging behind in terms of energy today, but the demands of your job or yo home duties may make it impossible to get the rest you need. |
| *For your body* | Keep your energy up with low-fat carbohydrate sources like fruit, a baked potato, a piece whole-grain toast, a smoothie, or a box of raisins. |

How I Feel _____

_____

My Thoughts _____

_____

## Day 100    Date _____

| Your baby today | Your baby's spine gets stronger every day so it can continue to support her growing body. |
|---|---|
| *For your baby* | Thanks to ultrasound imaging, you already have a photo of your baby. Why not put yo favorite ultrasound picture in a cute frame and display it on your desk at work or at home s you can gaze at your son or daughter all day? |

**our body today**

If you run your fingers down along the center of your stomach, you may feel the soft area where your abdominal muscles have started to separate.

**or your body**

Once the abdominal muscles separate to accommodate the growing uterus, they become more vulnerable to pulls and strains. Never do sit-ups while pregnant, be careful when lifting, and go slowly when getting up from a horizontal position. Your muscles will rejoin after birth, but your stomach may lose some of its tone.

*How I Feel*

*My Thoughts*

# Day 99    Date _____

**our baby today**

Your baby is gaining a special kind of fat in three key areas: at the nape of her neck, around her kidneys, and behind her breastbone. This "brown fat" is the same kind of fat that keeps hibernating animals warm in the winter. It will help your baby stay warm in the first few weeks after birth.

**or your baby**

Find out if the baby's father gets any paid or unpaid paternity leave benefits. If he'll need to use his vacation time when the baby comes, make sure he lets his boss know the approximate dates far in advance. If your husband or partner does not have the luxury of time off from work, start lining up some extra help from friends and family now.

**our body today**

By the end of your pregnancy, each of your breasts will have gained about a pound in fat and tissue for the purpose of breastfeeding.

**or your body**

If you buy nursing bras this early in your pregnancy, be sure to buy them at least a cup size larger. Your breasts will continue to grow as your pregnancy progresses and will increase in size again when your milk comes in. Choose a comfortable, breathable material knowing that you may wear your nursing bra to bed for extra support.

*How I Feel*

*My Thoughts*

Week 25 Weigh-in: _____ lbs

# Day 98   Date _____

### Your baby today

The last layers of your baby's retina, way in the back of her eye, have now finished formin

### For your baby

When decorating your baby's nursery, consider placing a mobile above the changing tabl Some babies dislike getting their diaper changed and being exposed to the cold air, so th visual distraction could prove handy. Bright, contrasting colors are the way to go, as thes are the first colors your baby can discern.

### Your body today

You may find yourself making long to-do lists of projects and tasks that need to be complete before the baby comes. You may be overwhelmed by all of the things you need to do prepare for your baby's arrival.

### For your body

Set realistic expectations for yourself and focus on the most crucial tasks at hand. Discussir your maternity leave with your boss, for example, is an essential task. Learn to let go of le: important projects like refinishing that nightstand to match the baby's crib. Enlist the he of others and avoid overextending yourself in these last few months of pregnancy. Rest essential to your baby's development and to your own wellbeing.

How I Feel _____

_____

My Thoughts _____

_____

# Day 97   Date _____

### Your baby today

Your baby's eyelids are no longer fused shut. He now opens them occasionally to observ the world around him.

### For your baby

Don't get lazy about taking your prenatal vitamins. Your baby still needs the extra suppo they provide. Set an automatic reminder on your computer or cell phone so you wor forget.

### Your body today

You are almost to the end of your second trimester! While the little aches and pains th characterize the third trimester are still ahead of you, they will be offset by the fact th you're drawing closer to the day you meet your baby.

### For your body

Keep up the good work, continue to eat healthy, and maintain a positive outlook. Tre yourself to a prenatal massage at a local spa today to reward yourself for the work you' done and raise a glass of sparkling lemonade to toast your baby's good health tonight.

How I Feel _____

_____

My Thoughts _____

_____

_____

## Day 96 Date _____

**our baby today**

Your baby now has working taste buds on his tongue and inside his cheeks.

**or your baby**

Some experts believe that your baby's food preferences are based, in part, on what foods he's exposed to in the womb. If you want a baby who eats all his vegetables, you'd be wise to start feeding them to him now.

**our body today**

If your blood pressure is too high, if you are diagnosed with preeclampsia, or if there is any threat of preterm labor, your doctor may place you on bed rest for the remainder of your pregnancy.

**or your body**

About 20 percent of women are put on some form of bed rest while pregnant. While staying in bed for weeks or months at a time can feel like a prison sentence when you're used to leading an active life, remember that you're doing it as a service to your baby. Rest can relieve the amount of pressure on your cervix and reduce contractions. It can also alleviate high blood pressure and increase the flow of nutrients and oxygen to your baby.

How I Feel _____

_____

My Thoughts _____

_____

## Day 95 Date _____

**our baby today**

Over the next month, the amniotic fluid that supports your baby's movements will decrease by about half. She'll have more room to move, but will not have the freedom of movement that a more watery environment provides.

**or your baby**

Drink a glass of orange juice today (preferably the calcium-fortified kind). The potassium it provides helps to regulate your baby's blood pressure and your own. It also offers a hearty dose of vitamin C and folic acid.

| Your body today | As the amniotic fluid in your uterus decreases, your belly becomes a captivating source of entertainment. Today the landscape of your rounded belly may change quite often as your baby kicks and twirls and pokes. |
|---|---|
| *For your body* | Take a warm bath today. If not for your own relaxation, do it to watch your belly dance as your baby moves around. Her activity level will most likely increase in the warm water—so much that little waves form all around you. |

How I Feel _____

_____

My Thoughts _____

_____

## Day 94    Date _____

| Your baby today | Your baby now sleeps for 20-30 minutes at a time, tossing and turning in the REM stages. It not known whether or not she dreams. |
|---|---|
| *For your baby* | Some women swear by the effectiveness of sound machines to drown out background noise and help their baby sleep after birth. Most of these machines offer a variety of newborn friendly sounds, including white noise and heartbeat settings. |
| Your body today | You may find yourself awakening easily at night and remembering more dreams than usual. |
| *For your body* | In the last few months of pregnancy, your sleep cycles change and you will probably experience more REM sleep than usual. This means you'll dream more and will stir more easily from sleep. Consider this Mother Nature's way of preparing you for the nighttime demands of caring for your newborn. |

How I Feel _____

_____

My Thoughts _____

_____

## Day 93    Date _____

| Your baby today | Your baby's lungs are maturing and as they do, she may endure recurring bouts of hiccups |
|---|---|

or your baby
When you go to purchase baby bottles, look for designs that prevent air bubbles from getting into the fluid. Some bottles are angled while others feature an air ventilation component. This will reduce gassiness and may ease colic (a term applied to babies who cry inconsolably, possibly from indigestion).

our body today
If you feel rhythmic or spasmodic motion in your stomach today, it is probably your baby dealing with a serious case of the hiccups.

or your body
The next time your baby has the hiccups, give your partner a chance to experience them. Place his hand on your belly so he can feel the rhythmic motions. Keep in mind that many of the pregnancy sensations to which you're accustomed are still exciting and new for him.

How I Feel

My Thoughts

# Day 92    Date

our baby today
Your baby is about 14½ inches long today from the top of his head to his heel.

or your baby
Considering buying a height chart to hang in your baby's room so you can mark his rapid growth.

our body today
You may experience some Braxton Hicks contractions today. If they persist, you may worry that you're going into labor.

or your body
Here are some indicators to help you distinguish between labor contractions and Braxton Hicks (false) contractions: False contractions are irregular and don't increase in intensity. They also tend to subside if you take a shower, lie down, or change position. Labor contractions follow a fairly regular pattern and grow in intensity. They are usually felt in the lower abdomen and radiate around to the lower back.

How I Feel

My Thoughts

# Daddy's Turn

Daddy's Thoughts and Feelings

Happiest 2nd Trimester Moments

_____

_____

_____

_____

_____

The Kind of Dad I Hope to Be

_____

_____

_____

_____

_____

A Message for My Pregnant Wife/Partner

_____

_____

_____

_____

_____

A Message to My Baby

_____

_____

_____

_____

_____

My Favorite Baby Names

# Day 91    Date _____

**our baby today**

Your baby now weighs about 2½ pounds, approximately one third of what her birth weight will be.

**or your baby**

If you decide to breastfeed, it may be difficult to determine how much milk your baby is actually getting. For this reason, some parents invest in an infant scale to track their newborn's weight gain at home to make sure it's progressing normally.

**our body today**

Congratulations! You made it to the third trimester—soon you'll be holding your newborn child in your arms. You have probably gotten used to your pregnant identity and the responsibilities that come with that role. You know exactly which cheeses to avoid, which fish to eat sparingly, and which foods give you the worst heartburn. You have already become the conscientious mother that your baby needs.

**or your body**

Your third trimester will bring a more immediate awareness of your baby, since her movements will be strong enough to distract you day and night. Knowing that your due date is just around the corner will force you to mentally prepare for life after baby. As much as you try to go about your normal life and work, your thoughts will inevitably return to the child you're about to meet. Allow yourself the freedom to daydream and the time to act on your "nesting" instinct and prepare your home for the little one.

How I Feel _____

_____

My Thoughts _____

_____

_____

# Day 90    Date _____

**our baby today**

Your baby's skin is red and completely covered in an oily, waterproof layer called vernix

**or your baby**

Try to put off buying things for your baby until after your baby shower. It will save you from having duplicates or having to return items later on.

**our body today**

Today, somebody may tell you that you're "huge" or that you look like you're going to give birth any day. You may occasionally glimpse your pregnant form in the mirror and stop to stare. Could that really be you?

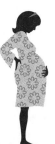

Week 26 Weigh-in:_____lbs

The best way to deal with the weight gain and body changes that happen in the next fe months to maintain some perspective—you won't look this way forever. Deflect an negative comments (as they are probably not meant to offend), but keep one ear ope when advice comes your way. You never know—it may actually be useful.

*How I Feel*

_____

_____

*My Thoughts*

_____

_____

> I had a client who told me, when he found out that I was pregnant, that he had thought I was getting "a little chunky." I was already in my third trimester by that time, and figured it was pretty obvious to everyone that I was pregnant, not chunky!
>
> —Mary G., mother of 5-month-old Sam

# Day 89    Date _____

**Your baby today**

Your baby's lungs are becoming more and more fine tuned, but they are not fully prepare to breathe air.

*For your baby*

If you are ready to buy crib bedding for your baby, you may want to leave the "bumper" the store shelf. A crib bumper is a long piece of cloth that lines the inside of the crib an prevents your baby's head from bumping into the rails. Because of concerns over suffocatic and SIDS (should the baby should roll into the bumper face-first), opt for the breathabl mesh kind or forego the crib bumper all together.

**Your body today**

Thoughts of delivering your baby vaginally may be causing you some anxiety. You have hea of women tearing or needing episiotomies to allow the baby to fit through the vagina.

*For your body*

Instead of worrying about what could happen on the day you deliver, empower yourself handle whatever comes your way. Do 10 reps of Kegel exercises today after reading th Squeeze the muscle you use to stop your urine flow. Hold for 10 seconds and release. [ this 10 to 20 more times to help build strength in the muscles around your vagina, anus ar urethra. It's commonly believed that consistent Kegel exercises leading up to birth can he you push the baby out and decrease your chance of needing an episiotomy.

# Day 88    Date _____

**Your baby today**    Your baby's hair is growing in on the back of his head.

**For your baby**    Baby bottles made from polycarbonate plastic contain the chemical bisphenol-A, also referred to as BPA. While the FDA is still investigating the potentially dangerous effects of BPA on infants, you may want to buy glass bottles for your baby or BPA-free bottles.

**Your body today**    If you're one of the lucky women who still enjoy frequent sex in the third trimester, take advantage! It's the perfect stress release for your body and a great way to stay connected to your significant other throughout the remainder of pregnancy. If you find that you're rarely in the mood, however, it could create some distance between you and your partner.

**For your body**    Assure your partner that you want to be close with him, but your pregnant body is just too preoccupied with other tasks. Enjoy a warm bath together, take turns giving each other massages, and come up with new ways to enjoy physical intimacy until your sex drive returns. Sometimes all you need to get your libido back is a little boost of self-assurance. Remind your partner that physical compliments will get him much further than pressure to have sex.

How I Feel _____

My Thoughts _____

**Your baby today**

If your baby is a boy, his testicles have descended into the scrotum. If your baby is a girl, h[er] labia have developed but will not come together to cover the clitoris until the last few wee[ks] of pregnancy.

*For your baby*

Until your baby's umbilical cord falls off (1 to 3 weeks after birth), a sponge bath is th[e] recommended method for cleaning him. This will help you keep the cord stump dry an[d] prevent infection. Lay him on a bath sling or a soft towel and use water and a mild soa[p] to dab him clean. Make sure your baby stays as warm as possible. Newborns do not nee[d] frequent baths—once a week should suffice. Bathing them too often could dry out the[ir] sensitive skin.

**Your body today**

You may find yourself grunting and groaning today as you get up from a soft couch, recline[r] or bed.

*For your body*

Some women use a birthing ball (a large plastic exercise ball) as a chair during pregnan[cy.] They balance on it while watching TV or talking on the phone to improve their posture an[d] alleviate minor backache and pain. During labor, a birthing ball can help support your bo[dy] in a squat position. If you kneel down and lean over the ball, you can rock your pelvis to he[lp] ease labor pains and to help the baby move into a better birthing position.

*How I Feel* _____

_____

*My Thoughts* _____

_____

As soon as I got to the hospital, my birth plan flew out the window. I wasn't interested in anything "alternative," like getting into creative labor positions. I just wanted to lie in bed and suffer through. They had to give me Pitocin, since every time I lay down, my contractions went away. It took twenty-four hours of labor before I was ready to push.

—Jennifer D., mother of 2-year-old Lana

**our baby today**   Your baby is gaining more baby fat and muscle today.

**or your baby**   You may lose some vitamin C content when eating canned foods like oranges, but overall frozen and canned foods retain their key nutrients. So, if you can't get fresh produce, make sure to at least buy the frozen or canned variety.

**our body today**   You may notice reddish-colored spider veins on your legs, face, neck, upper chest, or arms. Genetics and increased blood circulation are the most probable causes.

**or your body**   Crossing your legs can deter proper blood circulation and may promote or worsen the appearance of spider veins. Eating and drinking foods high in vitamin C (which keep veins healthy and pliable) can help to minimize them. While these branch-like markings should fade soon after delivery, stubborn ones may remain.

How I Feel _____

_____

_____

My Thoughts _____

_____

_____

**our baby today**   Your baby may hold his hand against his forehead for some length of time today. This is a fairly common fetal pose.

**or your baby**   The more fluids you drink, the greater your blood volume. The greater your blood volume, the easier it is to get essential nutrients to your baby. Try to drink at least 8 glasses of water, unsweetened juice, or milk every day.

**our body today**   You may be increasingly proud of your pregnant form and happy to receive some extra attention today.

**or your body**   Strut your baby bump with pride. Pull out the camera and take a few profile shots and belly close-ups so you can remember this unique physical state forever. Look back on older photos of your pregnant form to see how much it has changed.

How I Feel

My Thoughts

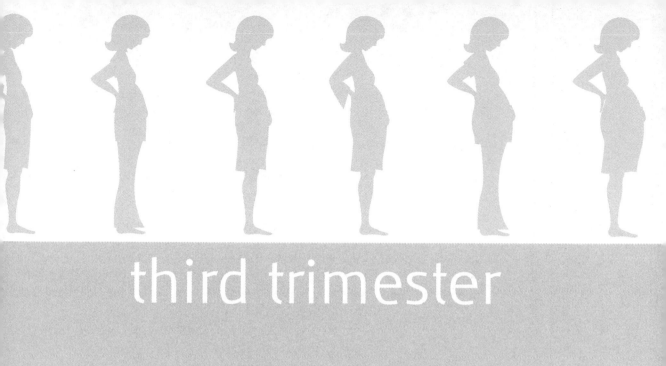

third trimester

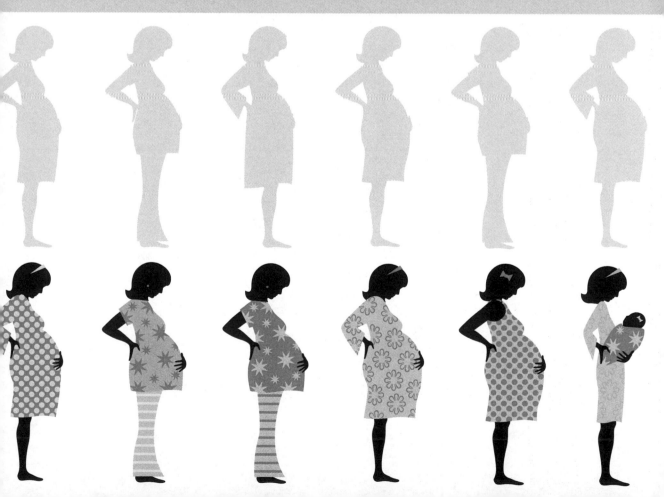

# Day 84    Date _____

**Your baby today**

Though it's getting harder to move around in your uterus, your little one can still stretch an kick. You will probably feel him kick at least ten different times this morning.

*For your baby*

Every day, your baby's bones require about 250 milligrams of calcium to develop and harde Keep up a steady supply of calcium so your baby doesn't need to borrow from your ow reserves. Three to four glasses of skim milk or orange juice will help you meet the dai requirement of 1,000 mg.

**Your body today**

Your weight gain is probably somewhere between 17 and 24 pounds.

*For your body*

If you notice a decline in your baby's activity level, let your medical provider know. She ca arrange for a nonstress test (a close monitoring of the baby's heartbeat) or a biophysic profile (a close monitoring of the baby's movements) to make sure that your baby is okay.

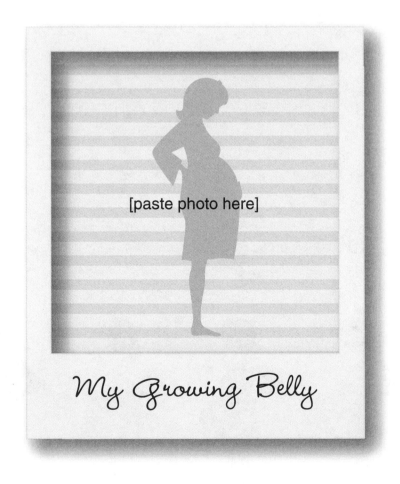

[paste photo here]

*My Growing Belly*

How I Feel

My Thoughts

## Day 83    Date _____

**Your baby today**
Your baby's brain is growing at a fast pace. The soft bones of his skull are designed to expand and make room for this growth.

*for your baby*
Take a nap!

**Your body today**
You will probably begin to see your healthcare provider every two weeks now that you are in your third trimester.

*for your body*
Be sure to write down any health concerns or questions that you may have before your prenatal appointments. It's easy to forget something in the short span of time you have with your provider. Encourage your partner to come with you to your next appointment so he can ask his own questions and become more familiar with the man or woman who is most likely to deliver his baby.

How I Feel

My Thoughts

## Day 82    Date _____

**Your baby today**
The previously smooth surface of your baby's brain has ridges and indents that reveal all the new nerve connections being built.

*for your baby*
Feed your baby the omega-3s his brain needs for healthy development. The best source of these fatty acids are cold-water fish like salmon, mackerel, sardines, and herring, but you can also get a fair amount of omega-3s from cooking with or using spreads with olive and canola oils.

Week 27 Weigh-in:_____lbs

**Your body today**  As your body readies itself physically for the job of childbirth, your mind may race with thoughts of your upcoming delivery.

*For your body*  If you haven't yet toured your hospital or birthing center, make sure that you arrange to do so. Becoming more familiar with the place where you will give birth (not to mention the route to take getting there) may put some of your anxiety to rest.

*How I Feel*

_____

_____

_____

*My Thoughts*

_____

_____

_____

# Day 81    Date _____

**Your baby today**  Your baby may open her eyes today, but only for a second or two.

*For your baby*  Even if you're desperate for a good tan, it's best to limit your sun exposure and avoid tanning beds until after the baby is born. Both can cause a significant rise in body temperature, posing a threat to your baby's health. While limited research has been done on self-tanning sprays and lotions, they are unlikely to penetrate your skin deep enough to pose a threat. Spray-tanning booths, however, are riskier because you can breathe in the chemicals.

**Your body today**  You may begin to notice some pronounced blue veins in your legs now or in the weeks to come. Chances are you have a family history of varicose veins.

*For your body*  Varicose veins are evidence that your body is working extra hard to pump an excess of blood through your body. You may feel discomfort or pain from varicose veins before you even notice them on your body. The best way to minimize or prevent them is to walk or exercise for about 30 minutes every day to help your blood circulate back to the heart. You may also want to use a stool to prop your feet when sitting for long periods of time.

*How I Feel*

_____

_____

_____

*My Thoughts*

_____

_____

_____

**Your baby today**

Your baby's brain is now more able to manage the tasks of breathing and body temperature regulation.

**For your baby**

If you want to determine whether your newborn baby is too hot or too cold, touch the back of her neck. If it's clammy and warm, she may be overheated. If it feels cold, she probably needs an extra layer or a warm snuggle. Don't judge by the temperature of her hands and feet, as these extremities run cold.

**Your body today**

At the end of the day today, you may feel completely run down and exhausted. Still, your mind is swimming with the tasks that need to be done at work and at home and you feel compelled to keep going.

**For your body**

Put down the mop, the laptop, the to-do list, or whatever else is keeping you from giving your body a much deserved break. Break plans with friends if you're just too tired. Prioritize your rest above all else for the next 80 days—your health and your baby's health is riding on your willingness to do so.

How I Feel _____

_____

My Thoughts _____

_____

**Your baby today**

Your baby is hearing, tasting, seeing and smelling better than ever today.

**For your baby**

Now that your baby can hear more sounds than ever, he may be growing accustomed to some of the louder noises in your home. Your dog barking, your vacuum cleaner, and the sound of your favorite television show may even be familiar to him by the time he makes his entrance into the outside world. Don't be surprised if, as a result, he can sleep easily through these sounds as a newborn.

**Your body today**

While no one may admit this to you, your usual gait may now resemble more of a waddle as your body adjusts to your extra weight and the loosened ligaments of your pelvic and leg joints.

**For your body**

Now that your body is moving in a different way, you may need to be more cautious of tripping and falling. The clumsiness of the third trimester is actually a blessing in disguise. Those "loose hips" that are making you wobble will also help ease the passage of your baby through your birth canal.

## Day 78 Date _____

**Your baby today**

The amount of tissue in your baby's brain has started increasing at a rapid pace.

*For your baby*

If you haven't yet picked a name for your little one, today is the perfect time to write dow some favorites and discuss them with your partner. If you need a baby name book to kic start the process, consider purchasing or borrowing one that groups names by category, lik *The Baby Name Wizard* by Laura Wattenberg. If you have already settled on a first name congratulations are in order. You've made one of your first difficult decisions as a paren Now you can shift your attention to finding a suitable middle name!

**Your body today**

You may exchange understanding smiles with another pregnant woman today at the ma the park, or the grocery store.

*For your body*

Make it your goal over the next few months to meet other expectant moms in your are Even if it means giving your phone number to someone you meet at the store, connectin with local moms online, or researching new mom groups in your community, your soci networking will pay off after the baby is born. A playdate with another new parent can be true lifesaver on difficult days.

How I Feel _____

My Thoughts _____

Gestational Week 28, LMP Week 3

## Day 77 Date _____

**Your baby today**

The full-body fuzz, or lanugo, that once coated every inch of your baby's body is starting rub off.

**For your baby**    If you haven't found a pediatrician for your baby, it's time to start looking. Ask your own doctors, family, and friends whether they have anyone to recommend. Most pediatric care offices will allow you to schedule a "meet-and-greet" with potential pediatricians. Some questions to ask include: 'How does this office handle after-hour emergencies?' and 'What length of time is allotted for regular appointments?' You may also want to find out whether their stance on breastfeeding, infant immunization, and prescription antibiotics (some feel that antibiotics are over-prescribed) are in line with your own.

**Your body today**    The ligaments in your body may be so relaxed that they cause your feet to spread out more. You may go up a whole shoe size and stay this way even after pregnancy.

**For your body**    There will be very few times in your life when shopping for a new pair of shoes is medically justified—this is one of them! Take advantage by splurging on a nice, comfortable pair to sustain you through the remainder of this pregnancy and beyond.

How I Feel _____

_____

My Thoughts _____

_____

_____

## Day 76    Date _____

**Your baby today**    Your child's skin is looking less wrinkled and she's growing rounder and chubbier every day.

**For your baby**    Pacifiers are a common tool for soothing babies, but many parents are hesitant to use them for fear that they could lead to nipple confusion (if the baby is not yet used to breastfeeding), a pacifier addiction that lasts well into toddler-hood, or the dreaded pacifier overbite. Other moms swear by the peace that a pacifier brings to their baby and their household and experience none of the repercussions mentioned above.

**Your body today**    You may notice that the mood swings of the first trimester have returned. One minute, you're crying over a cell phone commercial and the next you're yelling at your husband for using the wrong dishtowel.

**For your body**    The first thing you can do is to assure yourself that you're not losing your mind. Your mood shifts are most likely the result of pregnancy hormones, mounting anxieties as your due date approaches, and the nagging discomforts of the third trimester of pregnancy. One way to vent your frustrations is to go for a walk, enjoy some alone time, or meet up with an understanding friend.

Week 28 Weigh-in: _____ lbs

> My biggest worries right now are financial and logistical. Will we be able to save enough to support another person? Can we cut enough out of our budget so that I can stay home with the baby or work part-time? The cost of child care where I live is exorbitant and there are huge waiting lists for the best child care centers. I worry a lot about how it is all going to come together in the end.
>
> —LaRue, 4 months pregnant

*How I Feel* _____
_____
_____

*My Thoughts* _____
_____
_____
_____
_____

# Day 75    Date _____

**Your baby today**

Your baby's fingernails and toenails are completely developed and are growing in length.

*For your baby*

Don't forget to purchase some infant grooming items or add them to your registry. At first you won't need much more than a pair of miniature clippers for her little fingernails and toenails. Some baby nail clippers feature a magnifying glass or a large, easy-to-grip handle so you don't have to cringe with every snip.

**Your body today**

It may seem like your body is already stretched to the limit to fit that growing baby, but your uterus is determined to enlarge as needed. It will extend beneath your rib cage to keep up with the baby's growth.

*For your body*

Now that the top of your uterus is about 4 inches above your belly button, you may feel some strong kicks to your ribcage. Some of these kicks may be uncomfortable; some may even be a bit painful. Try shifting positions to encourage your baby to do the same. Avoid foods that seem to make your baby go wild, like very cold drinks or ice cream.

How I Feel

My Thoughts

# Day 74   Date _____

**Your baby today**

Your baby weighs about 3 pounds today and is over 15 inches long.

**For your baby**

As you get closer to your due date, you may want to consider your pain relief options during delivery. For most women, this means deciding between a natural, unmedicated birth (where breathing and other popular relaxation techniques are employed) or the pain relief option of an epidural. Over 50 percent of American women who give birth in a hospital have epidural anesthesia injected into their spinal cord area to decrease sensation in the lower half of their body.

**Your body today**

You have about a pint and a half of amniotic fluid in your uterus today. Every hour this fluid needs to be replenished with about a cup of water stored in your body.

**For your body**

Drinking lots of water during pregnancy helps to replenish the amniotic fluid in your uterus. It can also ward off hypertension, urinary tract infections, and even premature labor in your third trimester.

How I Feel

My Thoughts

# Day 73   Date _____

**Your baby today**

Your baby can follow a light source with his eyes today.

**For your baby**

When your baby is born, he will only be able to see objects clearly if they are within a few inches of his face. Be sure to hold him nice and close so he can experience seeing your face for the first time.

**Your body today**

You may find that your stomach is squished by the growth of your uterus and you feel full soon after you begin eating.

*For your body*  Eating large meals in the third trimester can leave you feeling uncomfortably full, bloated and wracked with indigestion. Stick with small meals—like a high-fiber cereal loaded with fresh berries.

How I Feel _____

My Thoughts _____
_____
_____

## Day 72    Date _____

Your baby today    Your baby's cerebral cortex is developing to support consciousness and memory. Things he hears and feels today may stay with him long after he is born.

*For your baby*    Now is a great time to narrow your lullabies down to a specific few. The more you sing a particular song, the more soothing and recognizable it may be outside the womb.

Your body today    Your rib cage has expanded by an inch or two so you can take in extra oxygen for the baby. This may cause you to breathe deeper than usual and may increase your overall lung capacity.

*For your body*    If you plan to breastfeed, now is a good time to shop for a nursing bra. Your rib cage is larger now than it will be when you're nursing, so shop for one that fits on the last hook setting. Remember to go up at least one cup size since your breasts will enlarge when your milk comes in.

How I Feel _____
_____
_____

My Thoughts _____
_____
_____

## Day 71    Date _____

Your baby today    The site where your baby's red blood cells are produced has shifted from her liver to her bone marrow.

*For your baby*    Your baby needs plenty of folic acid to grow and to continue making red blood cells. Pick your favorite green, leafy vegetable to incorporate into your diet today. A quesadilla with spinach (an abundant source of folic acid) and your favorite cheese makes a quick, vitamin-rich, mini-meal.

**Your body today**

By 3 p.m., you feel like your body has been sapped of all energy. You've been carrying the extra weight of pregnancy and sustaining your baby's development all day, but now you've hit a wall.

**For your body**

Grab a high-energy snack to get you through the toughest part of your day. A hard-boiled egg, a cup of yogurt, or a handful of almonds have the protein power you need to get your energy back.

How I Feel _____

_____

_____

My Thoughts _____

_____

_____

---

## Day 70    Date _____

**Your baby today**

Your baby will probably gain another half of a pound this week, reaching a total weight of about 4 pounds.

**For your baby**

Consider taking an infant CPR class this month. Knowing how to help your baby in an emergency can make you a more confident caregiver. Invite your partner to attend the class so he can be equally prepared should an emergency situation arise.

**Your body today**

Now is roughly the time when your coworkers or friends and family will hold a baby shower in your honor. If you don't love being the center of attention, an impending baby shower—especially a surprise one—can be a little nerve-wracking.

**For your body**

Keep in mind that family and friends want to celebrate your pregnancy and your growing baby. You'll need plenty of gear to get you through the first year, so relish in their generosity. If you are already well-equipped for baby's arrival, you may want to politely request an alternative type of baby shower. A baby book shower, for instance, invites guests to bring a favorite children's book to add to the baby's library.

How I Feel _____

My Thoughts _____

_____

Week 29 Weigh-in: _____ lbs

## Day 69    Date _____

**Your baby today**

Your baby's lungs and digestive tract are still in development, but the rest of her body is i full operation.

*For your baby*

There will probably be plenty of times in the next 68 days that you need an energy boost. I those moments, try to avoid the temptation to grab an energy drink. Many are loaded wit caffeine, herbs, and even chemicals that could do harm to your baby. Check the caffein content of anything you eat or drink and try to keep your daily consumption under 300 m Anything over that could increase your risk of having a low birth weight baby.

**Your body today**

Your breasts may leak a bit of colostrum today in preparation for nursing. If they aren leaking colostrum, don't worry. This is not a sign that your breasts are unprepared.

*For your body*

Ask your midwife or OBGYN whether they have a lactation consultant on staff to help yo address breastfeeding issues that arise after you leave the hospital. It may also be wise t generate a list of private lactation consultants and breastfeeding support groups in you area. Find out ahead of time what kind of help they offer, whether they will come to you home, and whether their services are covered by your health insurance.

*How I Feel* _____

_____

*My Thoughts* _____

_____

## Day 68    Date _____

**Your baby today**

There is now a hint of color in your baby's irises.

*For your baby*

Caucasian babies are normally born with grey-blue eyes that can change color up until th baby is about 9 months old. Darker-skinned babies usually begin their life with brown eye that may also get darker and deeper in color. The general rule is that newborns' eyes do n lighten, but they may darken over time.

**Your body today**

If you're already had your baby shower, you may be putting off the sometimes overwhelmin task of writing and sending thank-you notes.

*For your body*

Schedule time today to update all the addresses in your contact list in preparation fo sending thank-you cards. Print out two sets of address labels to make the process go mo smoothly. Why two sets? Remember that you'll receive a whole new crop of gifts when th baby arrives and you'll have even less time to send thank-you notes then.

## Day 67    Date _____

**Your baby today**    Your baby goes through restful and active (R.E.M.) sleeping stages throughout the day. Today he may only be awake with his eyes open for a few hours.

**For your baby**    Swaddling your baby is one way to help him sleep better. By wrapping him firmly in a light blanket, you can help him feel as though he is back in the warm confines of the womb. Swaddling also prevents his own startle reflex (which makes his arms and legs jerk suddenly as he sleeps) from waking him.

**Your body today**    Your bellybutton is probably close to "popping" at this point. If you have an "innie," your growing abdomen may have already stretched it into an "outie."

**For your body**    Plan on gaining about a pound a week over the next nine weeks. As your body gets bigger and more cumbersome, exercise may become less appealing. Resist the temptation to surrender yourself to the couch. Just thirty minutes of walking, swimming, or prenatal yoga can help you stay fit for delivery and will help balance out those inevitable late-night binges.

How I Feel _____

My Thoughts _____

## Day 66    Date _____

**Your baby today**    Your baby is getting a firmer grip every day. When he's born, he will be able to grab hold of you so tightly that you could almost lift him by the strength of his grip.

**For your baby**    If you've already acquired some clothes for your baby, be sure to wash them in a gentle, fragrance-free detergent before the baby arrives. Otherwise the clothes could irritate his sensitive skin.

| Your body today | Purple, pink, or brown streaks, the beginnings of stretch marks, may start to appear on your abdomen. Some may also appear on your breasts, hips, or thighs. About half of all pregnant women get these colored indentations in their skin when it's stretched to the limit. |
|---|---|
| *For your body* | You're in good company if you get stretch marks at this stage. If you don't see any yet, hold off on celebrating—stretch marks have a way of showing up in surprising places after delivery. No cream is proven to have a preventative effect, but it may make you feel better to keep the affected area moist or to apply a cream with vitamin E to improve its elasticity. Less than a year after you have your baby, these badges of motherhood will have faded significantly to blend in with the rest of your skin. |

*How I Feel* _____

_____

_____

*My Thoughts* _____

_____

## Day 65  Date _____

| Your baby today | If you are having identical twins, your babies may now grab hold of each other in the womb. At this point in the pregnancy, the growth rate of twins slows down, because the placenta can no longer sustain further growth and the babies are beginning to compete for nutrients. |
|---|---|
| *For your baby* | On average, most twin pregnancies last about 36 weeks. If you go into premature labor with twins, your medical provider's goal will probably be to delay your labor for a few more days so they can administer corticosteroids to the babies. These drugs will help your babies' lungs and organs mature more quickly to help support their survival outside the womb. |
| Your body today | Someone may tell you how "cute" your pregnant belly is today, but you may not feel that way at all. Indigestion may instead have you feeling uncomfortably bloated, full, or gassy after meals. |
| *For your body* | If you tend to drink seltzer or soda with your meals, try switching to regular water, milk, or tea. Don't lie down until at least an hour or two after you eat. If you still get indigestion at night, place some books under the back legs of your bed to keep your upper body elevated. Stacking pillows under your head and upper back can also help, but don't expect them to stay in place as you toss and turn in your sleep. |

*How I Feel* _____

_____

_____

*My Thoughts* _____

_____

**Your baby today**

Your baby is now able to turn his head from side to side to have a look around.

**For your baby**

As you design the nursery, keep in mind that your baby will quickly grow into a toddler. Rubber ducky wallpaper borders and pink bunny curtains may seem too babyish next year. To avoid having to redo the room later, don't get too specific with the décor. Stick with colors, shapes, and patterns that will grow with your child.

**Your body today**

Dinnertime and early evening can be a difficult time of day for a pregnant woman in her third trimester. You may find yourself too exhausted to pick up around the house, sort through the mail, walk your dog, or prepare a complete meal.

**For your body**

Allow yourself at least a half hour of rest before dinnertime or as soon as you walk in the door at night. Ignore the mess, the mail, and the kitchen until you have given your mind and body a little rest. (If you have other small children, this could prove difficult without the use of their favorite television show or some other distraction.) To ease the struggle of weekday meals, consider preparing a lasagna or casserole over the weekend when you have the energy. You'll have a few days' worth of meals to simply reheat.

**How I Feel** _____

_____

**My Thoughts** _____

_____

> I did prenatal yoga to stay healthy during pregnancy. I only did it once every two weeks or so, but I think it helped both physically and mentally. I also did a lot of walking.
>
> —Julie B., mother of 9-month-old River

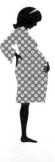

# Day 63     Date _____

**Your baby today**

Your baby's head is in proportion to the rest of his body. His arms, legs, and body ar getting chubbier.

*For your baby*

When you pick up your newborn, you'll need to support his head and neck with one hand He won't have any control over his head until he's at least a few weeks old.

**Your body today**

The layer of fat in your breasts has increased and you have significantly more milk glands t support breastfeeding. Little bumps may have appeared on the dark area surrounding you nipples. These are glands that secrete lubricating, antibacterial oil.

*For your body*

Your breasts are becoming full-fledged baby-nursing stations. They are even equipped wit a natural healing ointment for the soreness you may experience as your baby learns t latch. Massaging just a few drops of your own breast milk on your nipples will help sooth them between feedings, as will lanolin ointment made especially for nipple soreness.

How I Feel _____

_____

My Thoughts _____

_____

_____

# Day 62     Date _____

**Your baby today**

If your child is a boy, both of his testicles have now completely descended int the scrotum.

*For your baby*

Now is a good time to educate yourself about autism, a surprisingly common neurologica disorder thought to occur in about 1 of 250 births. Autism is four times more common in boy than in girls and can cause mild to severe impairment of social interaction and communicatio skills. For more information about autism, visit the Autism Society of America's website a www.autism-society.org.

**Your body today**

You may experience a sharp pain or cramp starting in one buttock and running down th back of your leg. This is called "sciatica" and it results from extra pressure being placed o the sciatic nerve in your lower back.

*For your body*

Avoid lifting, bending, or extensive walking as these can cause or aggravate sciatica pai Lie on the side that hurts or apply a cold pack if that seems to help. Taking it easy is one the best things you can do to alleviate nagging aches and pains.

How I Feel _____

My Thoughts _____
_____
_____

## Day 61    Date _____

**Your baby today**
Your baby is very active, kicking her legs and waving her arms. You might feel this more when you are lying down, because your movement likely lulls her to sleep.

**For your baby**
Dig into some omega-3-rich foods today to help facilitate your baby's brain development. Mix up a baby spinach salad complete with chickpeas and walnuts. Sprinkle on a dressing rich in canola or olive oil.

**Your body today**
Heartburn may strike again today, especially if you consume fizzy drinks, citrus fruits or juices, spicy, or fatty foods. You may find yourself popping antacids all day long to alleviate that burning sensation in your throat and chest.

**For your body**
Believe it or not, eating ice cream or drinking milk before a meal can help to coat your stomach and guard against heartburn. Dessert for heartburn relief? This may be the best news you've heard all day!

How I Feel _____

My Thoughts _____
_____
_____

## Day 60    Date _____

**Your baby today**
Your baby is probably in a head-down position right now. Her head may be pressing against your pelvic floor while her legs may kick under your ribcage.

**For your baby**
Write a personal message to your baby today. Use the "My Thoughts" section below to tell your child how excited or nervous you are to meet her and what kind of life you wish for her. When you're done, consider sharing your message with your partner and encouraging him to share as well.

Week 30 Weigh-in: ____lbs

**Your body today**

If you're like many women, fruit has been one of your top pregnancy cravings. If not, don' worry about it—a colorful array of vegetables can also give you the fiber and nutrient you need.

*For your body*

Grab a bag of ready-to-steam veggies at the supermarket today to go along with your mai course. They may be more expensive, but they'll be ready after just a few minutes in th microwave. Your aching feet and back will thank you.

*How I Feel*

_____

_____

*My Thoughts*

_____

_____

_____

_____

# Day 59    Date _____

**Your baby today**

Your baby is constantly breathing water into his lungs to prepare and strengthen them fo breathing air.

*For your baby*

If you're a vegetarian, your baby can still get all the protein he needs from a variety of dai products. If you're a vegan, you'll need to provide protein via a combination of whole grair and legumes. Four cups of brown rice, three cups of soy milk, a cup of tofu and a cup of sc yogurt can provide the protein your baby needs in a day.

**our body today**

The closer you get to your due date and the larger your belly grows, the more your baby-to-be will become a reality for your partner. You may find that he's suddenly talking and thinking more about your son or daughter.

**or your body**

Enjoy sharing in the excitement of a new baby with your husband or partner. Take advantage of the relative calm before the storm by spending lots of quality time together. Enjoy dining out and doing things that will soon become more complicated. Revel in the strength of your relationship, discuss how you will handle the relationship challenges that a new baby inevitably brings, and gush about the life-altering event that will soon deepen your bond.

*How I Feel* _____

*My Thoughts* _____

## Day 58    Date _____

**our baby today**

Your baby can probably distinguish the sound of one language from another and prefers to hear the language she hears you speak.

**or your baby**

Talking to your baby throughout the day will help her get to know your voice and learn your language. Consider reading your favorite children's book to her tonight before bed. If you do this every night until she's born, the familiarity of the story may relax her even after she's born.

**our body today**

You may have already decided that you will bottle-feed your child once she's born. Because breastfeeding is experiencing a surge in popularity, you may feel alienated by the overwhelming support of breastfeeding you read and hear about.

**or your body**

If you're one of many women for whom breastfeeding is not an appealing or practical option, look for support in other women who have chosen bottle-feeding. Bottle-feeding will allow you to involve your partner in a very crucial aspect of your newborn's care and give you more freedom to leave your baby with other people. Regardless of how you came to the decision to bottle-feed, trust in yourself to make the best decision for your child and surround yourself with as many supportive people as possible.

*How I Feel* _____

*My Thoughts* _____

**Your baby today**

Your baby can hear vowels more easily than consonants. For this reason, he may love all th "oohs" and "aahs" he gets as a newborn.

*For your baby*

Enlist someone to help you assemble your baby gear today. Strollers, cribs, bouncy seat and swings usually require some time and concentration to set up. Better now tha after the baby comes! You may also want to store up on batteries for all motorized gea Consider purchasing rechargeable batteries and a charger for items with music, lights, ar vibration—all of which drain a battery very quickly.

**Your body today**

At your next prenatal visit, your doctor or midwife may begin finalizing your birth plan wi you. She may want to know what kinds of medical intervention you are open to receivin whom you have chosen to join you in the delivery room, and whether or not you plan breastfeed.

*For your body*

If you want your husband or partner with you in the delivery room, begin discussing yo expectations with him. Let him know what kind of role you expect him to play. Do you wa him to massage your back during contractions or stand by silently for emotional suppor Do you want him to be your advocate ensuring that you're getting the best care possibl Will you be disappointed if he doesn't cut the cord? Communicating your wishes now ma alleviate your concerns as well as your partner's and make for a smoother delivery.

*How I Feel* _____

_____

*My Thoughts* _____

_____

**Your baby today**

Your baby's fast-growing brain has actually increased his head circumference by about 3 of an inch.

*For your baby*

Not sure whether you have enough clothing and apparel for your baby's first few month Four to five newborn outfits and a few packages of 0–3 month long-sleeve or short-slee onesies (depending on the season) should form the basis for his wardrobe. Eight to ten pai of socks and a few hats are a must for keeping baby warm in cooler weather. Buy a varie of socks or booties, as some will slip off baby's feet almost as soon as you slip them on.

**Your body today**

Your uterus is so enlarged that it is pushing your stomach and diaphragm up toward yo lungs. As a result, you may experience temporary shortness of breath or faintness.

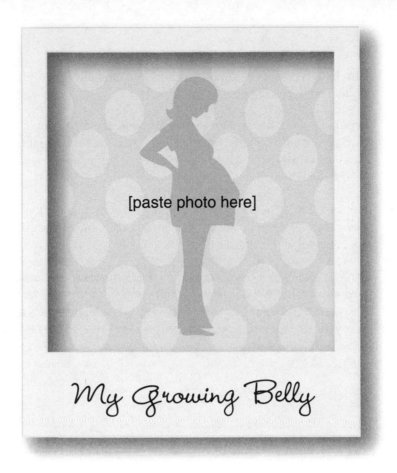

*My Growing Belly*

or your body Changing positions, moving more slowly, and sitting upright instead of leaning back should help to alleviate this sensation. Rest assured that your baby is getting enough oxygen even if you're short of breath.

tow I Feel _____

_____

My Thoughts _____

_____

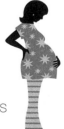

_____

Week 31 Weigh-in:_____lbs

## Day 55 Date _____

**Your baby today**

Your baby is beginning to store calcium, iron, and phosphorus to aid in the development his soft skeleton of bones.

*For your baby*

Your baby needs calcium to support his skeletal growth, but in order for you to absorb th calcium you eat, you need vitamin D. While dark-meat fish, eggs, fortified milk, and cod liv oil all contain vitamin D, just ten minutes of sun exposure a day can help you meet yo daily requirement.

**Your body today**

Many women fall out of love with pregnancy at some point. If you're fed up with your oversize body, physical aches and pains, and unwanted attention from strangers, remember why yo got pregnant in the first place.

*For your body*

For a definite pick-me-up, focus on all the things you look forward to as a parent. Think how much fun it will be watching your baby learn to smile, laugh, play, crawl, dance, ar talk. Imagine how good it will feel when he or she learns to kiss and hug you back. No matt how you feel today, tomorrow you're one step closer to the endless stream of rewards th come with being a mom.

How I Feel _____

_____

My Thoughts _____

_____

## Day 54 Date _____

**Your baby today**

Your baby is about 16½–17 inches long and weighs about as much as a bag of flo (4½ pounds).

*For your baby*

The average birth weight of a newborn in the U.S. is about 7½ pounds (girls tend to weig less than boys). In your baby's first week of life, he will probably lose 6 to 10 ounces of ext fat and fluid. After that, he should gain about 4 to 7 ounces every week.

**Your body today**

You may be experiencing a return of those first trimester pregnancy headaches. Thi trimester headaches are common and may be the result of poor posture or the physic stress of carrying around all that extra weight.

*For your body*

Chocolate, yogurt, peanuts, and cured meats are just some of the foods that tend to trigg migraines. Avoid them just in case. Be aware of how you're holding your body and try maintain good posture. If you need pain medicine, talk to your medical provider abo taking acetaminophen.

How I Feel _____

My Thoughts _____

## Day 53    Date _____

**our baby today**

Your baby's skin is changing from red and wrinkled to pink and smooth.

**or your baby**

If you're feeling stressed out today, take some time for yourself. Make an appointment for a manicure, call up an old friend, or enjoy an extra-long bath. A relaxed and happy mom makes for a healthy and happy baby.

**our body today**

You may be able to determine the position of your baby's body from the movements you can see and feel. His hiccups may tell you that his head and chest are down, while a series of strong kicks may reveal the location of his feet.

**or your body**

Don't forget to take a snapshot (or have your partner take a snapshot) of your very pregnant body this month. You may not feel photogenic at the moment, but you'll be surprised how much you'll enjoy looking back on the image years from now.

How I Feel _____

My Thoughts _____

## Day 52    Date _____

**our baby today**

Your baby may stick her tongue out several times today, a common behavior in babies of this age. She may be tasting the amniotic fluid, which changes flavor with the foods and drinks you consume.

**or your baby**

Most breastfeeding experts will advise you to wait 4 to 6 weeks after the baby is born to introduce the bottle. Any earlier and, they argue, you could undo the work you've been doing teaching her how to "latch" onto your breast. If you decide to stock up on bottles now, look for designs that mimic the shape of the breast and are meant to prevent nipple confusion.

**Your body today**

You may not be thinking about birth control at all right now, but after the baby comes you need a reliable form.

**For your body**

It takes your body about a year to fully recover from having a baby, so consider giving yourse at least that much time if you want to have more children. Whatever you do, don't fall fo the myth that breastfeeding is a foolproof method of birth control. It is true that you are les likely to ovulate or get your period until after you stop breastfeeding, but it's also impossib to know exactly when your body has regained its fertility. Using your period as an indicato of when you need birth control is taking a big risk.

*How I Feel*

_____
_____

*My Thoughts*

_____
_____
_____

# Day 51    Date _____

**Your baby today**

Today, your baby is better equipped to regulate her own body temperature.

**For your baby**

One of the things you should have in your home as soon as your newborn arrives is a rect thermometer. Rectal thermometers give the most exact temperature readings to help yo accurately determine whether your baby has a fever.

**Your body today**

You may have heard of an episiotomy before, but you're not quite sure whether it's a goo thing or a bad thing.

**For your body**

An episiotomy is a cut made to open the vagina wider during delivery. If your baby's hea is having trouble fitting through your vaginal opening on its own or if your medical provide needs to get the baby out quickly, he may numb the area and perform an episiotomy. If yo don't get an episiotomy, you may tear naturally on your own. Some medical providers prefe to let women tear on their own, as a tear may heal more quickly and is not as likely to exten toward the rectum. Discuss the procedure with your medical provider and find out his or he position on the issue.

*How I Feel*

_____
_____

*My Thoughts*

_____
_____

**ur baby today**

Your baby is growing steadily and will continue to do so even after her due date comes and goes.

**r your baby**

It may relieve you to know that most medical providers will induce labor if you haven't had the baby by 41 or 42 weeks (LMP). Babies grow at about a half a pound per week. Thus, the longer your baby stays in the womb after her due date, the bigger she will be and the more difficult it will be to deliver her vaginally.

**ur body today**

The top of your uterus should be about 5 inches from your belly button. You have probably gained between 22 and 28 pounds.

**r your body**

Don't be overly concerned if you are bigger than other women at this same stage of pregnancy or if you're gained more weight. Everyone carries their pregnancy differently and some women are prone to gaining more weight than others. Unless your medical provider is concerned about your weight, there's no need for you to be.

*tow I Feel*

*My Thoughts*

**ur baby today**

Your baby may open her mouth wide today in a big yawn. It's unknown whether these yawns indicate fatigue, boredom, or if they're just a stretching of the facial muscles.

**r your baby**

If you're looking to add more omega-3s to your diet to help your baby's brain development, look to grass-fed beef. Beef from grass-fed animals has about three times the omega-3 fats as the more prevalent grain-fed beef.

**ur body today**

Your belly button is probably a full "outie" by now. While some women see this as a milestone that they're almost ready to deliver, others are embarrassed by the visible protrusion.

**r your body**

If you don't like your belly button showing through your shirt or if the skin there is extra sensitive, cover it with a band aid.

How I Feel

My Thoughts

# Day 48    Date _____

**Your baby today**

Your baby's immune system is now equipped to help her fend off minor infections.

*For your baby*

Try to avoid taking your newborn to public places until she's at least a few weeks old. Th[e] more people to whom she's exposed, the more germs to which her undeveloped immun[e] system will be exposed.

**Your body today**

Your body is experiencing a peak in amniotic fluid at the moment, though this will chang[e] in a few weeks.

*For your body*

Educate yourself on the three different stages of labor so you can track how you'[re] progressing on delivery day. The first stage of labor is the longest (up to 20 hours). It sta[rts] when you feel real contractions and continues until the cervix has dilated to 10 centimete[rs]. This stage includes the active phase of labor (when contractions are about 5 minutes apar[t]. The second stage of labor usually lasts a few hours. It begins when the cervix dilates to [10] cm and ends when your baby is delivered. This is when the pushing happens. The thi[rd] stage of labor lasts about 5–30 minutes and includes the delivery of the placenta.

How I Feel

My Thoughts

# Day 47    Date _____

**Your baby today**

Your baby has sharp fingernails that have grown out to the ends of her fingers.

*For your baby*

Not sure how or when to childproof your home? You probably won't need ma[ny] childproofing products until your baby starts to get around on her own. Then you'll wa[nt] to cover at least the basics: Outlet plug covers, window blind cord shorteners (to preve[nt] accidental strangulation), cabinet and drawer locks, door knob covers (to keep children o[ut] of dangerous or unsupervised areas) and stair gates are some of the most crucial elemen[ts] for safeguarding your home.

**ur body today**

As your due date gets closer, your cervix will stretch and thin out before gradually opening to prepare for your baby's birth. In some women, the cervix may efface and dilate slowly over a period of weeks.

**r your body**

Your medical provider will check you in your last few weeks of pregnancy to feel if your cervix is effaced (0 percent effaced means it hasn't thinned out at all, 100 percent means it's completely effaced). During labor, dilation will be measured in centimeters. When you are 10 centimeters, your cervix is fully open and dilated. That means it's time to push.

*tow I Feel*

*My Thoughts*

## Day 46          Date _____

**ur baby today**

All of your baby's bones are hardening except for the ones in her skull which are soft enough to slide over each other. The pliability of her skull will help her pass through the birth canal in just 45 days.

**r your baby**

Most moms expect to bond with their baby as soon as they lay eyes on her. Don't be alarmed if you aren't consumed by motherly love in the first moments or days after delivery. Bonding is a process—for some it can take weeks or months of getting to know a baby before they experience that deep maternal connection.

**ur body today**

Sleeping becomes more challenging as a little thing like turning over onto your other side becomes a physical feat. You may pull an abdominal muscle trying to accomplish this seemingly simple task.

**r your body**

If you need help changing sleep positions or getting out of bed when you have to use the bathroom, consider waking your partner. If a friendly shove from a sleepy mate isn't your idea of a solution, consider purchasing some luxury bedding. Satin sheets and pajamas can help you slide around with greater ease.

*tow I Feel*

*My Thoughts*

Week 32 Weigh-in: _____ lbs

# Day 45    Date _____

**Your baby today**    Your baby's body is still covered in a fair amount of vernix, though some has rubbed off.

*For your baby*    If you don't already have a rocking chair or glider, put it on your "Must Have" list. Newborn have spent 266 days rocking in the amniotic waves of your uterus, so it makes sense that th surest way to soothe a newborn is by providing constant motion. Rocking chairs are great f this purpose, but a glider is usually more comfortable and resists sliding around the roo as you rock.

**Your body today**    As your growing baby puts more pressure on your bladder, constant trips to the bathroo become a part of everyday life. If you have a long commute to work, you may be forced add a bathroom stop along the way.

*For your body*    Don't deny yourself liquids in order to keep this bathroom habit in check. Do avoid caffeinate drinks, which make you have to pee more often.

How I Feel _____

_____

_____

_____

My Thoughts _____

_____

_____

_____

# Day 44    Date _____

**Your baby today**    Your baby is no longer floating freely in a pool of amniotic fluid. His movements a restrained, but still powerful.

*For your baby*    Up until this week, it was normal for your baby to assume all kinds of positions in th womb. Going forward, a baby in the breech position (head up, butt down) is more likely remain that way until birth. About 1 in 25 full-term babies assume the breech position. If a ultrasound shows that your baby is breech, your medical provider will take several facto into consideration (baby's size, pelvic shape, stage of pregnancy, etc.) before recommendir a C-section or vaginal birth.

**Your body today**    You may wonder why the shape and height of your bump are different than that of oth pregnant women you know.

The stronger your abdominal muscles were before pregnancy, the higher you will probably wear your baby bump. A first pregnancy may stretch out your muscles, causing you to carry lower the next time you're pregnant. Your bump may also look different depending on your baby's position in the womb: If he's facing your back, your bump may protrude more than if he is facing forward. A sideways-lying baby can make your belly look extra-wide.

How I Feel _____

My Thoughts _____

## Day 43    Date _____

ur baby today

Your baby may enjoy hearing classical music today, as its rhythm is similar to that of human speech.

r your baby

It's not too soon to look into local playgroups in your area. Not only will it be helpful for you to find moms you can compare notes with, but your baby may eventually benefit from observing and modeling the behavior of other children.

ur body today

While you may be rapt with love for your new little family member, don't be surprised if you are also overcome by emotion and exhaustion in the first few weeks as a new mom. Rapidly decreasing hormone levels and sleep deprivation cause about 7 in 10 new moms to experience some form of "baby blues" after delivery.

r your body

Your mind and body need time to recuperate from the overwhelming task of bringing new life into the world. Take all the help you can get in the first few weeks and don't forget to attend to your own needs as well as the baby's. Eat well, rest when you can, and treat yourself to a few precious moments of solitude when you need them. If depression lingers after the first few weeks of your baby's life and is characterized by thoughts of harming yourself or the baby or a general disinterest in the baby, you may have postpartum depression. Don't be afraid to admit these feelings to your medical provider and be sure to get immediate help.

How I Feel _____

My Thoughts _____

# Day 42 Date _____

**Your baby today**

Just as you are wondering how your body can accommodate any more baby grow, your baby is wondering the same thing. She's having an increasingly hard time getti around in there.

*For your baby*

If you have a dog or cat at home, you may want to take precautions before introduci your pet to your baby. Have someone present an article of your newborn's clothing to yo pet before you arrive home. That way, your dog or cat will at least be familiar with h scent when she arrives. Even if the actual introduction of pet and baby goes smoothly, avo leaving them together unsupervised.

**Your body today**

Today, you may turn some heads when you gasp or grab your belly after a strong moveme from baby. This can be slightly embarrassing in the midst of a work meeting or while checki out at the grocery store.

*For your body*

If the miracle of feeling your baby move has started to wear off, consider experiencing through someone else. Watching a close friend or family member (or your husband) lig up after feeling those jerks and twitches is a great reminder that there's something rare a beautiful going on inside you.

How I Feel _____

_____

My Thoughts _____

_____

_____

# Day 41 Date _____

**Your baby today**

Your baby's kidneys are completely developed by now. In fact, most of his body developed.

*For your baby*

If you haven't yet read up on breastfeeding, infant care, baby sleep training, C-sections, pai management techniques during labor, or any of the other big topics, now is a great tim Read key passages out loud to your baby so you can learn and bond at the same time.

**Your body today**

Starting this week or next, your medical provider will want to see you on a weekly basis.

*For your body*

If you haven't received a pre-registration packet from your medical provider, be sure to a for one at your next visit. If you arrive at the hospital in labor, it will save you from the diffic task of filling out paperwork in between contractions.

tow I Feel _____

My Thoughts _____

## Day 40    Date _____

**our baby today**

Your baby's liver is now starting to process waste.

**r your baby**

While it may be disturbing to think of your baby drinking in amniotic fluid, waste and all, his body is able to filter out the impurities. Those impurities remain in his intestines until the first 24 hours after birth. When this thick, green stool called meconium is finally passed, it as a reassuring sign that your baby's bowels are in good working order.

**our body today**

You may be one of the 10 to 30 percent of pregnant women with Group B streptococci bacteria, or GBS, in your system. Your medical provider may soon administer a vaginal and rectal culture to see whether you are positive for the bacteria.

**r your body**

This procedure is quick, painless, and crucial in preventing a major health risk to your baby. GBS in adults is not a serious concern, but a baby with GBS can more easily contract pneumonia, meningitis, or a blood infection. If you are positive for Group B strep, you'll be given IV antibiotics during labor to greatly reduce the chance of passing it on to your baby.

tow I Feel _____

My Thoughts _____

## Day 39    Date _____

**our baby today**

Your baby now takes up more space in your uterus than the amniotic fluid.

**r your baby**

Draft a baby announcement email today. Take the time to gather all the email addresses of those you wish to contact when the big day arrives. Save it in your draft folder so that all you need to do after your little one makes her debut is fill in the details (time of birth, weight, length, baby name), attach a photo, and hit send!

Week 33 Weigh-in:____lbs

| Your body today | The more walking and standing you did today, the more swelling you may have from blood pooling in your feet. |
|---|---|
| *For your body* | Take every chance you get to sit or lie down with your feet elevated. Wiggle your toes and rotate your ankles throughout the day to keep the blood moving. |

*How I Feel* _____

_____

*My Thoughts* _____

_____

# Day 38   Date _____

| Your baby today | Weight gain will be a big part of your baby's growth going forward. Today she weighs between 5½ to 6 pounds. |
|---|---|
| *For your baby* | Your doctor may order an ultrasound at the end of your pregnancy to check your baby's position in the womb and to estimate the approximate size of your baby. How much faith can you put in your medical provider's birth weight estimate? Experienced clinicians usually come within a pound of the actual birth weight by evaluating measurements taken during the ultrasound. |
| Your body today | If you feel less pressure on your diaphragm and more on your bladder, then your baby may have "lightened" (dropped down into your pelvis). |
| *For your body* | First babies usually drop a few weeks before their due date. Subsequent babies may not drop until the day their moms go into labor. |

> I went into labor early with my second son (two days before my scheduled C-section)! My husband and I were planning to organize the spare bedroom that long weekend . . . it didn't actually happen until a few weeks after I got home from the hospital.
>
> —Melissa D., mother of 2-year-old Aidan

How I Feel _____

My Thoughts _____

## Day 37    Date _____

**Your baby today**

Your baby is developing a more consistent schedule of sleeping and waking. She has four states of consciousness: active REM sleep, quiet sleep, active awake time, and quiet awake time.

**For your baby**

Shop around for birth announcements today if you plan on mailing them out after the baby is born. Gather mailing addresses and stamps now, because you may not have the time or energy after the baby is born.

**Your body today**

Your sleep schedule is probably getting more erratic as indigestion, leg cramps, and baby kicks keep you up part of the night.

**For your body**

Believe it or not, you may be more comfortable sleeping on a couch or recliner at this point in your pregnancy. They do a better job of keeping your upper body comfortably elevated as you sleep.

How I Feel _____

My Thoughts _____

## Day 36    Date _____

**Your baby today**

Antibodies for all the various diseases to which you are immune are now being passed to your baby through your bloodstream and amniotic fluid.

**For your baby**

To protect your newborn from germs, it's best to wash your hands often when caring for him. Don't be afraid to ask friends and family members who come to visit to do the same.

**Your body today**

If you're having a C-section, your hospital stay will probably be about 4 days. A vaginal birth usually requires 2 days of hospitalization.

*For your body*    If you're a planner, chances are you've already lined up help for when you get home fro[m]
the hospital. Don't forget to also line up childcare (if you have other children) or a pet sitt[er]
for the period of time you'll spend in the hospital.

*How I Feel* _____

_____

*My Thoughts* _____

_____

_____

# Day 35    Date _____

**Your baby today**    Your baby has probably grown to the length he'll be when born, somewhere between 18 a[nd]
20 inches.

*For your baby*    Consider buying a molding kit that allows you to make, preserve, and/or frame his ti[ny]
handprints and footprints soon after birth.

**Your body today**    As your baby gets bigger and bigger, it may be harder to imagine birthing him vaginally.

*For your body*    If you're concerned about tearing during a vaginal delivery, there's some evidence th[at]
massaging your perineum (the skin between your vagina and rectum) with pure vegetab[le]
oil from now until your due date can help minimize tearing. A midwife or birth attenda[nt]
may also be able to massage your perineum as your baby is being born to help preve[nt]
excess tearing.

*How I Feel* _____

_____

_____

*My Thoughts* _____

_____

_____

# Day 34    Date _____

**Your baby today**    Your baby has lost most of the soft hair that once covered his body and much of the wa[xy]
coating of vernix that protected his skin.

It's recommended that you hold off on applying sunscreen on your baby until he's at least 6 months old (because of the sensitivity of newborn skin and the unknown effects of sunscreen chemicals on infants). This doesn't mean you can't take your new baby outside. When you do, just make use of items like clip-on or built-in canopies, car window shades, wide-brimmed sun hats, and full-coverage clothing to provide the necessary sun protection.

One thing you may not miss about life before pregnancy is having a monthly period. Once your baby is born, your body will begin to bleed again as if you are having a menstrual period. This is your body's way of getting rid of excess blood, uterine tissue, and mucus. It can continue for 2 to 6 weeks.

Prepare for heavy postpartum bleeding by purchasing heavy flow pads. Bring some to the hospital and keep some at home. While you may prefer tampons, their use is discouraged due to risk of infection.

How I Feel _____

_____

_____

My Thoughts _____

_____

_____

Day 33     Date _____

Your baby may break a smile in the womb today, but that smile probably won't return until 4–6 weeks after he is born. Smiling is one of the few behaviors that babies perform in utero and stop performing at birth.

Life outside of the womb will be a difficult transition for your child. You can ease the transition by simulating the environment of the womb as best as possible. Limit visitors in her first few days as she adjusts to life outside, provide continual warmth and comfort, and speak to her in a gentle, soothing tone. Carrying her close to your body in your arms or in an infant sling and providing constant motion (rocking, walking, and light bouncing) can also help comfort her in the days and weeks following birth.

Braxton Hicks, or false contractions, may strike with greater frequency now.

To prepare for true labor, find out how close together your contractions should be before heading to the hospital. Most medical providers advise laboring at home until contractions are roughly five minutes apart.

Week 34 Weigh-in: _____ lbs

## Day 32    Date _____

**Your baby today**

Your baby's face is plump and smooth today. If she has a raised birthmark, it is probab[ly] already visible.

*For your baby*

Some birthmarks are thought to be a skin abnormality resulting from displaced cells in th[e] first trimester of baby's development. Others are caused by a collection of blood vesse[ls] under the skin. About 80 percent of babies will have some sort of distinguishing mark [at] birth. It's not always easy to predict whether the mark will fade or remain for life.

**Your body today**

You may already be thinking ahead about how you're going to work off all th[e] baby weight.

*For your body*

Expect to lose about half of the weight you have gained immediately after birth. Losing th[e] rest will take some patience and commitment. If you have a C-section, you will need to gi[ve] your body at least six weeks to recover from surgery before engaging in exercise other tha[n] walking. Those who deliver vaginally can begin exercising sooner.

## Day 31    Date _____

**Your baby today**

Your baby has just a few more days to rotate into a head-down position for birth.

A baby who remains in a breech position beyond this week can sometimes be manually flipped through a procedure called an "external cephalic version." If this procedure is recommended, a doctor or specialist will attempt to physically coax your baby into a head-down position. It is a fairly uncomfortable procedure for the mom and most likely for the baby (whose heart rate will be closely monitored throughout), but it is often successful.

Today, a plug of mucus protects your tightly closed cervix.

One sign that your cervix is opening and that you are at least within a few days (or possibly at the start) of labor is the passage of the mucus plug through your vagina. You may or may not notice this plug, often tinged with blood, when it passes.

How I Feel _____

My Thoughts _____

# Day 30  Date _____

While your baby's development is nearly complete, she would still be considered pre-term if she were born today. She is not considered full term until 38 weeks from your last menstrual period.

About 1 in 10 U.S. babies is born preterm. Preemies tend to have more health issues at birth and may have long-term behavioral, learning, vision, hearing, and breathing issues. The earlier the baby is born, the greater the risk of her having these issues. If you think you are going into labor early, bring it to the immediate attention of your medical provider. When caught early, premature labor can often be brought to a halt.

You may start to feel huge and awkward as you carry 25–35 pounds of extra weight into the final weeks of your pregnancy.

Try to remember that the longer your baby stays inside your body, the healthier she will probably be at birth.

How I Feel _____

My Thoughts _____

# Day 29    Date _____

## Your baby today

Your baby is putting on a lot of weight in these last few weeks. From now on, she will ga
about an ounce a day.

## For your baby

Just as you may not look your best after labor and delivery, give your newborn some time f
her true cuteness to emerge. The trauma of delivery may leave her face puffy and swolle
and her head slightly cone-shaped after being pushed through the birth canal. Planne
C-section babies are an exception to this rule: they tend to look truer to form after deliver

## Your body today

Long walks may become less appealing as your body gets harder to lug around and swolle
feet and ankles cause discomfort.

## For your body

Even if it's a short walk, a stroll here and there can help get your blood circulating, keep yc
in better shape for delivery, aid digestion, and improve your mood.

How I Feel _____

_____

_____

_____

_____

My Thoughts _____

_____

_____

_____

_____

Gestational Week 35, LMP Week 3

# Day 28    Date _____

## Your baby today

Today, your baby may have a full head of dark, light, or red hair up to an inch long! Do
expect him to have the same hair color as you or your husband, because you're a
to be surprised.

## For your baby

You may automatically decline a second cup of coffee, a delicious-looking soft cheese, o
glass of wine today. Looking out for your baby's health has already become second natu
Take pride in the sacrifices you have made so far in pregnancy. They are a strong indicati
that you'll be a great parent to your child.

## Your body today

If you've been cautious with your diet and have cut back on habits like smoking and drinkir
then your body is probably healthier now than ever.

Use the momentum of pregnancy to carry on these healthy habits long after your baby is born. Many women begin practicing healthier eating and lifestyle habits after their first pregnancy. Just as your baby deserves the best nutrition and health you can offer, so does your own body.

How I Feel _____

My Thoughts _____

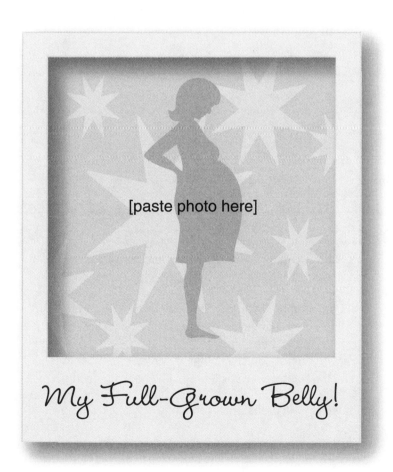

My Full-Grown Belly!

Week 35 Weigh-in:_____lbs

Your baby today    Your baby is about 19 inches long and weighs over 6 pounds.

*For your baby*    If you'll be working after the baby comes, solidify daycare plans with your chosen provide
Put down a deposit, arrange for your baby's start date, and fill out any necessary forms.
ease your stress when you go back to work, consider arranging a daycare "test run" a fe
weeks before your return date. Drop off your baby for just a few hours to help you and yo
baby adjust to the new arrangement.

Your body today    You may wish you didn't have to bring your child to daycare at all, but feel as though you ha
to due to financial need or because you've invested so many years in a successful career.

*For your body*    Consider the option of watching another child while you stay home with yours. It may bri
in enough money to allow you to care for your own child full or part time—if that's somethi
you want to do. Whether you choose a family member, a daycare provider, or you stay hon
with your child, have confidence that you've made the right decision for your family. The
is no one right answer.

How I Feel _____

_____

My Thoughts _____

_____

Your baby today    Your baby is getting ready to breathe outside the womb, and her lungs are already coated
a material called surfactant which helps them expand.

*For your baby*    Don't be alarmed if you notice that your newborn's breathing is noisy and irregular in t
first few weeks. (The more premature the baby, the longer it will take for her breathing
regulate.) Many a new mom loses sleep obsessing over every choke, gurgle, and pause
breath. If you find yourself doing the same, remember that her new lungs need time to wc
out all the kinks before she'll breathe in an even rhythm.

Your body today    Your weight will probably stay roughly the same from now until you deliver.

*For your body*    Collect take-out menus from a variety of local restaurants. You may be too busy or tired
fix meals for yourself after the baby comes, but keeping up your energy will be crucial. Y
may also want to stock up on store-bought frozen foods or make your own meals and free
them for later.

How I Feel _____

My Thoughts _____

our baby today
Many experts believe that labor begins with a signal from your baby. If so, secretions from his adrenal glands may soon kick-start your labor.

or your baby
Keep taking your prenatal vitamins, even though you may feel like you've already done all you can to support your baby's growth. Your body can still benefit from the nutritional boost these vitamins provide. If you breastfeed, your medical provider may recommend that you continue taking them until you stop breastfeeding.

our body today
The amount of amniotic fluid in your uterus is on the decline. When you give birth, there will probably only be about 2 to 6 cups of fluid remaining.

or your body
Have someone take a few close-up photos of your belly today. Your giant middle may be unremarkable to you at this moment (after nine months of watching it grow), but one day you'll be amazed to see exactly how your body looked holding your child.

How I Feel _____

My Thoughts _____

our baby today
Your baby's development has slowed down significantly, but his weight gain is steadily advancing.

or your baby
Before you can even leave the hospital with your baby, you need to have the baby's rear-facing car seat installed in the back of your car. Today may be a good day to read the installation instructions and give it your best shot. If you're not sure whether you've strapped it in correctly (it's more complicated than you think), you may want to get a car seat safety check at your local police or fire station.

| Your body today | Up to 25 percent of your current weight gain can be attributed to water retention. |

**For your body**  To keep the discomfort of swelling and bloating to a minimum, avoid eating processed and salty foods as they tend to make the problem worse. Eating dried fruits, bananas, and other foods high in potassium can help alleviate swelling.

*How I Feel* _____

_____

_____

*My Thoughts* _____

_____

_____

# Day 23   Date _____

**Your baby today**  Your baby's immune system is getting even stronger today.

**For your baby**  Your baby will receive many vaccinations in her first year of life to protect her from a variety of serious and life-threatening illnesses. Recent controversy regarding vaccines and autism has caused some parents to question whether the benefits of infant immunization outweigh the risks. For more on the issue, visit The American Academy of Pediatrics' website at: http://www.aap.org/advocacy/releases/autismparentfacts.htm.

**Your body today**  Your image of childbirth may be similar to the one often portrayed in movies and television. A woman lying flat on her back to labor and push. If you've taken a child birthing class, you may already know that there are a number of other positions used to facilitate labor and enable delivery.

**For your body**  Squatting is one of the best methods for fitting a baby through the pelvis once the cervix is fully dilated. It opens your pelvis up to 30 percent wider than if you were to lie down while pushing. Practicing the squat position while you're still pregnant will strengthen your leg muscles so you can hold the position during delivery. Enlist your birth partner to help support you in a squat today so you can both practice getting comfortable in this position.

*How I Feel* _____

_____

_____

*My Thoughts* _____

_____

_____

# Day 22    Date _____

**Your baby today**

Congratulations: Today your baby is full-term! This is an important milestone since it means her lungs are fully developed and she's ready to live and breathe outside the womb.

**For your baby**

Breathe a sigh of relief knowing that there is every reason to think she'll be healthy when she's born. Kudos to you for carrying your baby to this advanced stage of development!

**Your body today**

Today you may look back on your journey through pregnancy and feel a great sense of accomplishment and relief that you're almost to the finish line.

**For your body**

Tonight, celebrate your accomplishments by treating yourself to a movie marathon of comedy films about pregnancy. Some options include *Juno*, *Knocked Up*, *Baby Mama*, *Nine Months*, and *Father of the Bride, Part II*.

**How I Feel** _____

_____

_____

**My Thoughts** _____

_____

_____

# Day 21    Date _____

**Your baby today**

Eighty percent of babies arrive within two weeks of their due date. Yours could be readying himself for his arrival as you read this.

**For your baby**

If you haven't yet washed your baby's crib or cradle bedding in a gentle detergent, it's time to do so.

**Your body today**

While your baby could come anytime in the next few weeks, you may be stressed knowing that you still have plenty of work to finish at your job before the baby comes.

**For your body**

In case you do go into labor before your due date, it's best to start wrapping up work obligations now. Get your boss and/or your replacement up to speed on any ongoing projects, organize your work area, and write down the location of any important items or files. Write up a summary outlining the status of your work if you think it will help. That way, others can easily pick up where you leave off.

Week 36 Weigh-in: _____lbs

## Day 20      Date

**Your baby today**      Your baby has developed powerful sucking muscles in her cheeks.

*For your baby*      Wash newly purchased nursing bras, pacifiers, and bottles to prepare for yo
baby's arrival.

**Your body today**      Late pregnancy discomforts may make you wish you could stop working as early as today.

*For your body*      If medical issues related to your pregnancy (such as carpal tunnel syndrome, sciatica,
prescribed bed rest) are preventing you from being able to do your job, you may be ab
to take unpaid leave under the Family and Medical Leave Act. For more information, go t
http://www.dol.gov/elaws/esa/fmla/faq.asp.

How I Feel _____

My Thoughts _____

## Day 19      Date _____

**Your baby today**      If your baby is head-down, she may push off the wall of the uterus with her legs until h
head gets jammed down into your cervix. This means your baby has "dropped" into her fin
birth position.

*For your baby*      Your baby won't need much in her first few days spent at the hospital. Pack a few newbo
outfits or onesies, including one special outfit for her first photo shoot. A newborn pacif
(if you plan to use one), an extra swaddling blanket, an infant sling if you have one, and
3-month outfit in case you give birth to an extra-large baby may also deserve a spot in yo
hospital bag.

**Your body today**

You may experience a burst of energy today just thinking about the excitement that lies ahead for you and your family.

**For your body**

Put that energy to good use and pack your bag for the hospital! Some things you may need for your own comfort in the hospital are: your favorite pillow, soothing music, a camera and some extra batteries, a comfortable nightgown and robe, some early maternity clothes to wear home from the hospital (or stretchy, non-maternity clothes with elastic waistbands), and nursing supplies like bras, nipple-soothing lotion, a breast pump, and—if you have one—a breastfeeding support pillow.

How I Feel

My Thoughts

---

# Day 18        Date

**Your baby today**

Today your baby weighs about 2 billion times more than when he was a simple, fertilized egg.

**For your baby**

You will be working hard in the coming weeks taking care of your newborn as he adjusts to the outside world. While the reward for this effort may not be immediately felt, all the dirty diapers and sleepless nights will be worth it the first time he smiles at you.

**Your body today**

You may be more in love with your husband or partner now than ever as you both wait to meet the child you have made together.

**For your body**

While sex is not always an easy feat this far along in a pregnancy, intimacy can still be a part of your relationship. If you find that you don't have the energy for sex, find other creative ways to spend time together. Now is a great time to see a movie or go out to dinner, because it will be a lot more challenging in a few weeks!.

How I Feel

My Thoughts

## Day 17   Date _____

**Your baby today**

Your baby's waistline measurement is now just a little bit bigger than the circumference of his head.

*For your baby*

If this is your first child, you may want to buy a book about your baby's first year of development. Pediatricians aren't always available for all the little questions that crop up as your baby grows. Every new parent needs an objective resource to consult as her child ventures into new stages and reaches new milestones. There is a wide variety of books available, so ask your friends for recommendations or check out Amazon.com.

**Your body today**

Your nipples may be extra sensitive and your breasts may still be a bit sore as they continue to change and grow.

*For your body*

Ignore anyone who advises you to attack those sensitive nipples with a loofah to prepare them for the rigors of breastfeeding. This is no time to be inflicting more pain and discomfort on yourself. Count on your nipples to toughen up on their own if need be and maintain a positive outlook: some women don't feel any pain while adjusting to breastfeeding.

How I Feel _____

_____

My Thoughts _____

_____

_____

_____

## Day 16   Date _____

**Your baby today**

Your baby has acquired about 15 percent body fat by now.

*For your baby*

To reduce the risk of SIDS, avoid over-bundling your baby. As a rule, an infant will need one more layer of clothing than you would to be warm. Keep in mind that if you sleep beside them, they will need less clothing as your body temperature will raise theirs considerably.

**Your body today**

First-time moms, women over 40, women whose sisters and mothers had preeclampsia, and women carrying multiples all have a higher risk of preeclampsia.

*For your body*

If you're at higher risk for preeclampsia, be on the alert for symptoms like severe and persistent swelling, blurred vision, severe headaches, abdominal pain, and infrequent urination. Not sure what kind of swelling is questionable? Obvious swelling in the face and hands that doesn't go away is more indicative of preeclampsia than swollen hands and fingers that resolve themselves when you rest.

How I Feel

My Thoughts

# Day 15     Date _____

**Your baby today**

Your baby's lungs and brain are the only organs that have not yet fully matured. They will function well enough at birth, but will continue to develop long after.

**For your baby**

Warming up a bottle in the microwave can leave hot spots that could burn your baby's mouth. Heating up a bottle on the stove takes time, more than you've got patience for when the baby's crying for his middle-of-the-night feeding. If you decide to bottle-feed your baby, there's no reason why you can't serve him cold or lukewarm baby formula. Mix a few bottles before bed every night so you can simply grab one out of the fridge and go when the baby cries.

**Your body today**

The muscles at the top of your uterus are incredibly strong. During each contraction, they are as forceful as a 55-pound weight pushing your baby down through the birth canal.

**For your body**

While it's much easier said than done, the best way to manage contractions of this intensity is to relax your body as much as possible. Long, deep breaths will help you get enough oxygen and stay relaxed. Short, rapid breathing can make you light-headed and work you into a panicked state.

How I Feel

My Thoughts

Week 37 Weigh-in:____lbs

# Day 14    Date _____

**Your baby today**

Today your baby has more bones than you. Some of his 206 bones will later fuse together as he grows.

*for your baby*

The doctor or midwife who delivers you may ask if you want to see your baby's head (in a mirror) as you push him through the birth canal. Those who say 'yes' may find it highly motivating to see that they're only a few good pushes away from meeting their children.

**Your body today**

You may feel unusually cranky today as you field phone calls and emails asking if the baby has come yet.

*For your body*

If you're having a lot of Braxton Hicks contractions or if you expect to deliver your baby early, these last few weeks of pregnancy can be torture. Do what you can to distract yourself from the pregnancy and the baby: Read up on current events or celebrity gossip, email an old friend, re-organize your kitchen cupboards—whatever it takes to keep your mind off the subject today.

How I Feel _____

_____

My Thoughts _____

_____

_____

# Day 13    Date _____

**Your baby today**

Your baby has developed a vast range of reflexes by now. He has over seventy different physiological reactions to outside stimulus.

*For your baby*

Immediately after birth, your newborn's response to stimulation, muscle activity, heart rate, skin color, and ease of breathing will be evaluated and rated on a 1-10 scale. This Apgar score is used only to determine whether further observation of your baby is needed. Any score between 7 and 10 is considered normal.

**Your body today**

If you're having a planned C-section, it may be scheduled for this week!

*For your body*

Recuperating from major surgery is a challenge when combined with caring for a newborn. Arrange for at least two weeks of help after your surgery. It will take at least that much time to return to driving a car or carrying anything heavier than your baby. Arrange a place to sleep on the first floor of your home so you can avoid climbing stairs for your first few days home.

## Day 12    Date _____

**Your baby today**

Today the placenta is losing its efficiency at providing nutrients to your baby. Its crucial role in sustaining your baby's life and growth is coming to an end.

**For your baby**

Your breast milk may soon take over the role of the placenta in supporting your baby's ongoing growth and providing enzymes and hormones that enhance your child's development.

**Your body today**

You have about 14 to 16 milk ducts in each breast that carry milk to the nipple. If you notice some wetness when you take off your bra, those ducts are already at work transporting colostrum (the precursor to breast milk) to your nipple.

**For your body**

If you decide to breastfeed your newborn, you may actually feel your uterus contracting as you do so. Oxytocin—a hormone emitted during breastfeeding—helps your uterus shrink back to its former size and minimizes your postpartum bleeding.

## Day 11    Date _____

**Your baby today**

Your baby's heart and arteries are capable of transforming to help your baby breathe air. Their structure alters as soon as he takes his first breath. This change enables them to pump blood to your baby's lungs.

**For your baby**

If you haven't yet settled on a full name for your baby, finalize a list of the top three to take with you to the hospital. Sometimes the baby you imagine as you're selecting names looks strikingly different than the one staring up at you on delivery day. Give yourself the freedom of a few names and you're more apt to find one that fits.

| Your body today | Diarrhea or nausea may be a sign that birth hormones are clearing out your body in preparation for labor. |
|---|---|
| *For your body* | The best foods to eat when gearing up for labor are the same foods you would eat before a marathon. Complex carbohydrates like pasta provide the lasting energy you'll need to keep your strength during a long labor. |

How I Feel _____
_____
_____

My Thoughts _____
_____

## Day 10    Date _____

| Your baby today | Your baby is still building up the temperature-regulating layer of fat beneath her skin. |
|---|---|
| *For your baby* | If your baby's health is in question at this stage, your medical provider may suggest inducing labor. Some of the most popular reasons for inducing labor include placental abruption (the placenta separating from the uterine wall), preeclampsia, gestational diabetes, dangerously low levels of amniotic fluid, and risk of infection from your water breaking prematurely. |
| Your body today | The estrogen, oxytocin, and prostaglandin levels in your body are on the rise. These hormones are relaxing the ligaments in your pelvis and are adding elasticity to your vaginal tissues. |
| *For your body* | Make sure your husband or birth partner understands the various phases of labor as well as any pain management techniques you plan on using. The more confident and knowledgeable he feels about the process of labor and delivery, the better he'll be in supporting you through it all. |

How I Feel _____
_____
_____

My Thoughts _____
_____

## Day 9    Date _____

| Your baby today | Your baby is building a store of new skin cells today to replace the outer layer of skin he's now shedding. |
|---|---|

**For your baby**

Have fun trying out all your baby gear today so you can work out the kinks ahead of time. If you've purchased a baby monitor, add some batteries and test the sound/visual transmission with the help of your partner. Figure out how to fold and unfold your stroller, practice attaching your infant car seat to the car seat base or stroller, and pull out your infant sling to see how it adjusts for comfort.

**Your body today**

You may have a hard time seeing your pubic area well enough to groom it at this point in your pregnancy.

**For your body**

Don't worry about how your privates will look to the nurses, midwives or doctors during labor and delivery. Not only have they seen it all, but they have much more important things to focus on while assisting your birth than the upkeep of your pubic hair.

How I Feel

My Thoughts

# Day 8    Date _____

**Your baby today**

Your baby boy or girl probably weighs over 7 pounds today!

**For your baby**

Many babies outgrow their extensive newborn and 0-3 month wardrobe before they've had a chance to wear every item. A big baby is even more likely to zoom quickly through those early sizes. If you suspect that you have more baby clothes than you'll need, wash and fold your favorites before the baby arrives and keep the tags on the rest. That way, you can exchange unworn baby outfits for something in a larger size.

**Your body today**

You may start to feel frustrated if your physical limitations prevent you from doing everything you want done before the baby arrives.

**For your body**

Make your rest a priority as it will make you more prepared to deal with the work of labor. As much as you may want to run errands, clean your house, or hang wall decorations in the nursery, enlist your husband or close friends and family to help you with household chores and preparations for your baby's arrival.

How I Feel

My Thoughts

## Day 7    Date _____

**Your baby today**

The soft spots on your baby's head mark the gaps between her yet-to-be-fused skull bones. These gaps reduce the circumference of her head by up to one inch, helping her fit through the birth canal more easily.

*For your baby*

Soft spots make all new parents a little nervous. Rest assured knowing that there is more than just a layer of soft skin between your baby's brain and the outside world. A tough fibrous membrane offers considerable protection at each soft spot until the skull bones fuse. The soft spot at the back of your baby's head will close in a few months while the one at the top of your baby's head will usually close up between 8 and 18 months of age.

**Your body today**

You may feel something leaking today and wonder if you're urinating or your water is breaking.

*For your body*

Only about 1 in 10 women experience a heavy flood of water when their water breaks. Usually, it's a slow trickle that feels suspiciously like peeing. If you're questioning whether your water has broken, call your doctor or midwife immediately so he or she can check to see if the amniotic sac has ruptured. This may be the start of labor!

How I Feel _____

_____

My Thoughts _____

_____

_____

## Day 6    Date _____

**Your baby today**

Your baby is enjoying his last days in the balmy, 100-degree climate of your womb.

*For your baby*

Placing your newborn against your body immediately after birth will give him the warmth he craves and will help ease his adjustment to the colder, harsher atmosphere of the outside world. Don't be surprised if your baby immediately roots for your nipple and wants to feed.

**Your body today**

You may wake up today hoping it's the day you'll meet your baby and end up frustrated when the day comes to a decidedly uneventful close.

*For your body*

While you can certainly try, it's almost impossible to think of anything but the baby at this point in pregnancy. Since you need to keep busy and you're probably thinking of your child anyway, write a letter to your baby or film a video diary where you and your partner can share your excitement about meeting him.

## Day 5        Date _____

**Your baby today**    Your pregnancy hormones have caused your baby's scrotum or vulva to swell.

**For your baby**    If you believe that birth rates coincide with the lunar cycle (or if you just need something to do while waiting for the baby to come), you may want to check the lunar calendar today to find the next full moon.

**Your body today**    While there is no scientific proof relating birth rates and the cycle of the moon, many labor and delivery nurses will attest that their patient rate increases around the time that the moon becomes full.

**For your body**    Labor is called "labor" for a reason, so rest as much as you can in preparation.

## Day 4        Date _____

**Your baby today**    The remnants of your baby's slippery vernix coating combined with the stream of fluid that comes when your water breaks may help your baby slide out of the uterus.

**For your baby**    If you do receive an epidural during labor, aim to have it "wear off" by the time you need to push. If you can't feel what's happening from the waist down, it may be difficult to know when to push and how to do so effectively.

**Your body today**    Today your contractions may seem to regulate and get closer together before disappearing entirely.

Week 38 Weigh-in:_____lbs

*For your body*

If you are having a lot of contractions but are not yet in labor, walking can sometimes help get the process moving. Don't try to cover too much ground, though, or you'll be spent before you get to the most physically demanding part of giving birth.

How I Feel _____

_____

_____

My Thoughts _____

_____

## Day 3          Date _____

Your baby today

Your baby will soon exchange his watery breaths for gulps of air and his 1-room studio for a seemingly endless world of wide-open space in which to move, grow, and learn.

*For your baby*

Unless your doctor supervises or advises you otherwise, avoid trying to self-induce labor. Nipple stimulation, castor oil, sex, certain herbs, and spicy food are all rumored methods of stimulating contractions, but some can cause intense, lengthy contractions that limit the transmission of oxygen to your baby.

Your body today

You may be conflicted knowing that pretty soon, your body will be your own again. While shedding some of the weight and discomfort of pregnancy and having more freedom to eat and drink what you want may be appealing, you may also know that you'll miss the days when your baby was all yours.

*For your body*

Up until now, pregnancy has allowed you to experience a unique and magical connection with your baby—a connection that no one else will ever share. As a new mom, you have the opportunity to build upon that connection to form an even stronger relationship with your child as you get to know him and watch him grow up.

How I Feel _____

_____

_____

My Thoughts _____

_____

_____

_____

## Day 2          Date _____

Your baby today

Thanks to pregnancy hormones, your baby's breasts may be swollen and slightly enlarged.

**For your baby**

Don't be dismayed if you notice that a few drops of milk leak from your baby's nipples in the first few days after birth. This is a strange but harmless effect of pregnancy hormones.

**Your body today**

You are more than ready to meet your baby today!

**For your body**

If you haven't already stopped working, it's now time to slow things down considerably and focus on your upcoming job as a new mom. Don't venture too far from home as you await the beginning of labor and keep your cell phone charged and ready in case you need assistance.

*How I Feel* _____

_____

*My Thoughts* _____

_____

_____

## Day 1        Date _____

**Your baby today**

Today, your baby may emerge from your body and let out her signature birth cry. The sound is so unique that it distinguishes her from every other child in the world. When you hear this cry, you know that your baby's life has truly begun and that yours has changed forever.

**For your baby**

Whether your baby arrives today, tomorrow, or in two weeks, she will be well worth the long wait. Don't be afraid to spoil her in the first few weeks and months after she's born. She will need as much love and human contact as you can provide to grow and flourish.

**Your body today**

You've finally arrived at Day 1—the official end of your pregnancy! You have spent a whopping 266 days dedicated to the little life inside you and your reward is about to come. Your body has hosted the greatest miracle there is, and for that it deserves the utmost respect and admiration.

**For your body**

Take one last look at your pregnant form in the mirror, because it will soon fade into a memory. Take a photo to record this image forever. Look back on the journey you have traveled to get here and describe some of the most wonderful and most difficult moments you experienced along the way. One day, when your baby is grown, this journal will bring you back to the true beginning of your relationship.

*How I Feel* _____

_____

*My Thoughts* _____

_____

_____

# My Birth Story

Date and time labor started: _____

The weather that day: _____

What my contractions felt like: _____
_____

How I coped with labor contractions (pain medications, birthing props, positions, etc.):
_____
_____
_____

How my partner handled the labor: _____
_____
_____

Length of my labor: _____

My labor story in my own words: _____
_____
_____
_____
_____

My Baby

Date and time of birth: _____

My baby's name: _____

Why we chose the name: _____
_____
_____

My baby's weight: _____

My baby's length: _____

My baby's most striking features: _____

Who my baby looks like: _____

What I thought when I saw my baby: _____
_____

Other details about my baby: _____
_____

# Helpful Books and Websites

The American College of Obstetricians and Gynecologists. 2000. Planning Your Pregnancy and Birth, 3rd ec Washington, D.C.: The American College of Obstetricians and Gynecologists.

American Pregnancy Association, http://www.americanpregnancy.org

Aron, Elisabeth, M.D. 2008. Pregnancy Dos & Don'ts. New York: Random House.

BabyCenter, http://www.babycenter.com

Campbell, Stuart, M.D., 2004. Watch Me Grow! New York: St. Martin's Press.

Flanagan, Geraldine Lux, 1996. Beginning Life. New York: DK Publishing.

Sears, William, M.D. and Martha Sears, R.N. 1997. The Pregnancy Book. Boston/New York: Time Warner Boo Group.

Shulman, Martha Rose and Jane L. Davis, M.D. 2002. Every Woman's Guide to Eating During Pregnancy Boston: Houghton Mifflin.

theBump, http://www.thebump.com

# About the Author

Aimee Chase is a freelance writer living in the Boston area with her husband and son. Her favorite thing about pregnancy are ultrasounds and ice cream binges. Her least favorite things are leg cramps and nause. that just won't quit. She wrote this book while counting down the days to the birth of her second son.

# Index